Coping with Aging Parents

CHRIS GILLEARD

AND

GLENDA WATT

With a Foreword by
Dr Magnus Pyke

Published by Macdonald Publishers, Edinburgh
Edgefield Road, Loanhead, Midlothian EH20 9SY

The authors and publishers are
grateful to Age Concern for their
help in preparing this book.

Printed in Scotland by
Macdonald Printers (Edinburgh) Limited

Foreword

We live today at a time when science is predominant. There is no place on earth so distant that it is out of reach of our telephone. And as we gossip with our grandmother and ask her what the weather is like in Sydney, we think little of the great machines which were used to raise up into its orbit around the earth the satellite that transmits our words. We accept it as commonplace that every problem is soluble by science. Are there not microchips to form the core of the computers governing the robots which man the factories? Cannot video-tapes capture the sight and sound of each passing moment, freeze the instant and play it back to allow us to relive the past?

Our attitudes to health and medicine are the same. Within little more than the last half-century, scientific medicine has, it would seem, done away with the infectious diseases which once used to kill young and old indiscriminately. We no longer expect to die from pneumonia, typhoid, cholera or tuberculosis (the once insidious consumption), while smallpox has been extirpated from the face of the earth. In a society such as ours, science has increased the expectation of life and continues to do so. Is it surprising that we come to believe that there is no ill for which scientific knowledge cannot provide the remedy? Yet we know, when we stop to think, that even though we can with growing confidence expect to live to be old, yet no matter how successful medical science becomes, the overall death rate will remain unchanged at 100 per cent. And those of us who take thought are also aware that, even though medical knowledge has provided great benefits—for example in the treatment of diabetes, some aspects of cancer, and Parkinson's disease—knowledge is never complete. The goal of those who work on problems of the old, of health throughout life until the moment of death, is still to be attained. There are some fortunate people who cope well with the physiological changes which inexorably accompany the aging process right up to the moment of death. More often, however, advancing old age is accompanied by incompetence, ill-health, humiliation and decay. Thus, the burden of looking after old parents can be a heavy one.

Dr Gilleard and Glenda Watt have written a practical manual to help those on whom such a burden falls. Perhaps the main weight is the unceasing responsibility. Young couples with new babies quickly come to realise that, night and day, their duty is to keep watch, to be on hand, to do what needs to be done. But gradually the load lightens. In

Contents

Foreword

ten or twelve years, the children are growing up and part of the watchfulness can be relaxed. With aging parents the responsibility is reversed. It is no heavy duty—quite the reverse—to visit one's old mother once a week. But when the responsibility involves a constant watch, 24 hours a day, seven days a week, over a confused old woman who, in her bad moments, shows no gratitude or understanding, it is then that the ordeal—seemingly never-ending—is great. It is then that the authors' list of organisations, some official and some voluntary, from whom the caring son or daughter can ask advice will prove its worth. Oh that it could tell where a good friend prepared to take over every Wednesday (let us say) could be found! The main part of the book gives, just as its title implies, sensible information about all those topics of which the life of an aging invalid is composed— forgetfulness, incontinence, constipation, lack of appetite and contrariness, quite apart from the more dramatic incidents of stroke, dementia, accident and death.

For those who care, part of the problem is not knowing what lies ahead. The authors describe what may happen and how it can be faced. From time to time, when the problems seem too much for common sense, they say that a doctor's help should be enlisted. The special knowledge he possesses may enable him to solve the problem. Yet the doctor, playing his part, as the son and daughter are playing theirs, soon comes to know that there are—as there always will be— things he does not know, and when he can only do the best he can. This book helps those who are called to look after their aging parents to do the best *they* can.

Magnus Pyke
London, March 1983

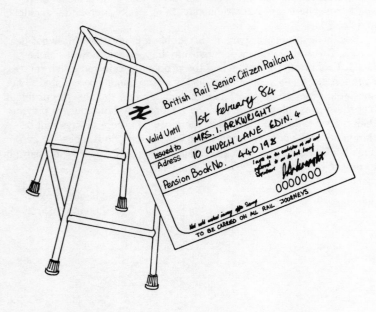

Which represents old age?

1 What is 'Old'?

You, the reader, may well be over the age of 60, yet you probably do not consider yourself an old person. The passage of time and your own aging are by no means parallel processes. You may notice that your muscles are less strong, your joints less flexible, and recovering from colds and other illnesses takes longer than it used to: you may receive a pension, and travel or go to the theatre at special 'senior citizen' rates. But these experiences do not lead you to feel old: you may feel your body growing older, yet inside you are aware of the continuity in your life, that everyday sameness which does not feel like age. It is the restrictions of infirmity, not age, which present the real challenge.

This book, therefore, is addressed as much to those over 60 as to the under-60s. Not only daughters and sons, but brothers, sisters, husbands and wives may each be faced with the challenge and the responsibility of caring for someone for whom age has brought infirmity or disability.

We will use the terms infirmity and disability to refer to those restrictions in the ability to carry out activities of daily life without assistance from others.

Many 70- and even 80-year-olds are the carers, not the cared for. We hope that this fact will gain increasing recognition in a society which tends to equate 'old' with 'infirm' or 'disabled.' Indeed we hope that as many readers will turn to this book to seek help for their husband, wife or sister, as will turn to it to seek help for their father or mother.

For most people, becoming old is experiencing having an elderly body. Inside, we are aware of the continuities in our life, the common threads of life and experience which hold together our childhood, working life and retirement. Our body may grow old, and refuse to perform the tasks we once expected from it: to some extent most people accept this fact, perhaps with regret, perhaps with contentment. Each year of life adds to our experience, and we may be aware of the growth that is always taking place. For many people in their 70s, however, each year also takes something away—a step that is less springy, a sense of tiredness that comes more easily, a growing awareness that the machinery of the body is less reliable than it once was. These two processes, of growth and decline, are not matched even in the same person, let alone between people.

Sometimes decline may seem to be uppermost; a winter of ill-health can make us feel old. Our experience may be one of losses, personal and physical. At other times, growth may be the more evident. Grandchildren going to college, discovering a forgotten friend, planning a holiday, visits from a distant son or daughter. More often perhaps, life continues with a comfortable sameness and we can lose ourselves in everyday activities which bring their own satisfactions. At such times, there seems no need to question the passage of time, nor to reflect upon old age.

But while our own life may give few clues of approaching age, others close to us may seem to be changing. We may spot the signs of old age and find ourselves becoming conscious of the changes and growing disabilities of those close to us (be they husband or wife, brother or sister, father or mother). This may be a slow process, one that we adapt to little by little, or it may, perhaps more often, be a sudden change, brought on by an illness or a fall or behaviour that seems out of place. Such changes are often associated with a change in circumstances, such as a holiday, moving house, or widowhood. We suddenly become aware that our relative is not his or her usual self.

From this point on, it may seem as though things gradually go into decline. Disability may become more and more prominent. More and more time may be spent in caring and worrying. It is unfortunate that many people rarely have the opportunity to discuss with others just what problems they are faced with, in looking after the elderly disabled. Often it is a task which seems more and more to isolate the duty of caring onto the shoulders of one particular person. Sometimes this is accepted as natural—a wife may feel it is her duty to care for her disabled husband, a son may feel it is his duty to care for his elderly disabled mother. Other family members may seem to have enough on their plate, or have difficulties of their own. Such isolated caring may be your choice, but it may also seem to be imposed and you may feel very much left on your own to shoulder the responsibility. We have prepared the checklist opposite to help you identify the level of disability for the person you are looking after, to help put your situation in perspective.

Check your answers to each of the following questions. For each NO, score 1 point. For each 'with difficulty' score ½ point.

What is 'Old'?

	Yes, no difficulty	Yes, but with difficulty	No, needs help
Can he/she do shopping without help?			
Can he/she walk outside without help?			
Can he/she get into and out of bed without help?			
Can he/she dress and undress him/herself without help?			
Can he/she use the toilet without help?			
Can he/she get in and out of a chair without help?			
Can he/she wash his/her hands and face without help?			
Can he/she take a bath without help?			
Can he/she feed him/herself without help?			
Can he/she cut his/her toenails without help?			

0 points is zero disability. 10 points is maximum disability. Scores of 1-3 represent moderate disability, where there may be a need for some formal help, such as a home help or visits from a chiropodist. Scores of 4-6 represent moderately severe disability, where the extent of caring imposes more strain than many can cope with. Scores of more than 7 are extremely rarely found; if you are caring for someone whose disability is in this last range (very severe disability) you are doing an extremely demanding job, and should try to take advantage of all the help available to you.

Coping with Aging Parents

It may be not so much a question of physical disability that causes concern, but more the behaviour we observe. Personality and character are rarely altered by age—though it is perhaps true to say that as we grow older, we become generally less nervous and less impulsive. Often, the concerns of the world become less intense and attitudes tend to be less passionately held than in younger adult years. A 'difficult' elderly relative is likely to have been a difficult person to get along with even when younger and a 'demanding' person is similarly likely to have exhibited such traits throughout their adult life. Major personality change is unusual and a sudden change in habits— e.g. a normally meticulous, houseproud person becoming careless and indifferent to her house and personal appearance—is usually a sign of illness, rather than 'aging.' Some elderly people are particularly prone to depression, especially those who have always had a pessimistic view of their achievements, and of the world generally.

There are certain stresses that are particularly connected with old age. Retirement, widowhood, loss of income and loss of friends, episodes of illness which are harder to recover from, all these are an increasing feature of our experience as we grow older. Reactions to these stresses vary from denial and apparent disregard, to a sense of hopelessness and helplessness. The older person may protect him or herself from the effects of such potential stresses by 'disengaging' from an external concern for the world or by devoting much attention to one particular area of interest, be it a hobby such as gardening ('he lives for his allotment'), or the immediate family ('she dotes on her grandchildren'), or on their health (he's obsessed with his bowels'). Alternatively, especially in the youthful period of the 60s and 70s, the person may seem to be expanding his interests, becoming involved in voluntary work, the Church, local politics, travel. Another 'style' of adjustment is the more placid 'rocking chair' strategy, where the elderly person becomes content to be looked after, making little active demands upon life, and enjoying a relaxed, supported existence. Whatever strategy is adopted, even if it is an aggressive independence from others, it is important to recognise that adjusting to the stresses of old age involves continuity. We do not become different people when we reach 65 or 70 or 75. The more our lifestyle links together the past, present and future, the more likely we are to be well adjusted.

What is 'Old'?

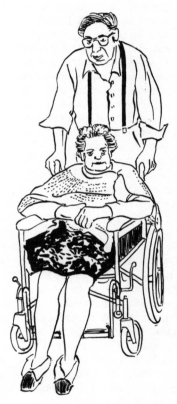

Many carers are themselves over 60

Coping with Aging Parents

A crabbity old man is not easily changed and if that has always been his way, then he will be better adjusted to facing stress by being allowed to remain crabbity. Caring for difficult members of the family needs acceptance and patience and a respect for the consequences of each life as it develops over the years. We may want to make our sister less fussy, our husband less domineering, our father less complaining, but we must recognise that if someone has survived and managed 60 or 70 years with particular characteristics, then those characteristics have proved their value, to the individual at least.

To sum up, let us recognise that aging is something that we are more likely to observe in others, rather than in ourselves. Aging, biologically, represents a change in the vulnerability of the body, an increased difficulty for the various tissues and organs to respond when things go wrong—through infection, damage, stress or accident. Disability reflects the meeting of biological aging with external forces that disrupt our everyday physiology, to which our bodies cannot adequately respond. The consequence is a restriction, a degree of handicap that impedes, but rarely totally prevents our maintaining a view of ourselves as still the same person, the same self which we were and which we all wish to remain, the sum of our unique life experience. Psychologically, on the other hand, aging is simply the growing awareness that we are not immortal, that the self which we have built up over the years can be challenged, can be faced with a variety of physical assaults. We need to accept that with increasing years, we must give due recognition to our physical health, to remain as fit, physically and mentally, as we can. Should we still be faced with disability, we need to recognise that such changes, however radical, do not mean that we must abandon our previous view of ourself, nor should such changes lead us to give up.

The biggest fear of many of the elderly is that of senility, when the rule of self over self, is broken, and mental control is lost. Aside from that devastation, loss of adequate control of a limb or an eye, even of the bladder is something that we all should be capable of accepting, should it occur. However much we revise our view of what we can do we can remain essentially the same person throughout most of the disabilities that are linked with old age; this task is made easier by others' recognition of our self's continuity in the face of the physical changes we may suffer. That is the most important message for all those, elderly or not, who support and care for an infirm old person.

2 An A,B,C, of Services

The single most important source of support for an elderly infirm person is the family. Since the ultimate goal of caring is to help the elderly person to maintain physical and mental functioning at as full a potential as possible, it is only right that the family's efforts should be recognised, complemented and sustained by both statutory and voluntary organisations. All too often community resources are unavailable or inaccessible to elderly people and their families. Problems of access and availability occur particularly in rural areas, where services are spread too thinly to give the support needed. However, there is still a general ignorance about the services that do exist, and the benefits to which many carers are entitled. The main aim of this chapter is to provide carers with information about services and benefits, and to suggest an approach to the care of the elderly disabled person which involves rationally managing and sharing that care amongst the various support systems.

The first step is to make as objective an evaluation of the person's needs as possible. This can be done within the family or between members of the family and professionals (GPs, hospital services, social services, etc). How great is the disability? What are the main problems? Is the disability temporary or permanent? Can it be prevented or will it worsen? What assistance is required in day-to-day living?

The second step is to identify the care and support that is available. This will include immediate and distant family members, friends, neighbours and organisations with which the elderly person has had contact—including the church, ex-workmates and colleagues—and finally, community agencies, both statutory such as the GP, health visitors, home nursing services, and social services, and voluntary, such as Age Concern and local Voluntary Services Organisers.

The third step is to identify one key person from each of these three areas of support who is prepared to act as the principal helper, and who can most effectively deliver support and assistance, drawing upon others in their area. Finally, the co-ordination of these three support systems—family, neighbourhood and service organisations— can be undertaken to enable the elderly person's needs to be met as adequately as possible. The idea of a 'primary care manager' is that he or she can ensure that the maximum assistance is given with the minimum burden imposed on any one individual.

Thus, a daughter may take on this role for her mother, who is disabled, but still lives with her husband. The daughter may arrange for her father to have a break, by taking her mother home for short periods. She may arrange with her sister to come in on alternate Sundays to help make lunch. Together with the GP, she may press for a home help to be provided. A district nurse may come in to give the mother an all-over bath once a week, social services may provide an incontinence laundry service, arrangements may be made for the father to visit, and be visited by, members of the local church or ex-workmates while a volunteer or other family member 'granny sits' for an afternoon or evening. By these means, the daughter is able to visit occasionally with most of her time free to be spent with her own family yet reassured that her mother's main needs are being attended to.

To be most effective in such a role, you must be fully aware of the numerous services that exist. While it is unfortunately true that many services which exist on paper are not locally available, it is even more the case that services which *do* exist locally are often not known to the carers. In the list that follows we have included national organisations as well as locally organised services, since they can very often provide helpful advice and useful information. We hope that you will find this guide a useful aid that can answer some, if not all, of your questions.

ACCIDENTS

Royal Society for the Prevention of Accidents, Carron House, The Priory, Queensway, Birmingham 4.
021-233 2461.

Branch address: Royal Society for the Prevention of Accidents, 41 South West Thistle Street Lane, Edinburgh EH2.
031-226 6856.

This organisation gives information and advice about the prevention of accidents in the home. The Environmental Health Officer and Health Visitor will also give advice about home safety.

An A.B.C. of Services

AGING

Age Concern: England, Bernard Sunley House, 60 Pitcairn Road, Mitcham, Surrey CR4 3LL.
01-640 5431.
Age Concern: Scotland, 33 Castle Street, Edinburgh
EH2 4DN.
031-225 5000.

Provides advice, information, training and development services for those working with, and for, elderly people; and for elderly people themselves. Age Concern campaigns nationally for elderly people. There are many local branches—look for their address in the telephone book.

Age Concern: Wales, 1 Park Grove, Cardiff CF1 3BJ.
0222 371566.

Age Concern: Northern Ireland, 128 Great Victoria Street, Belfast BT2 7BG.
Belfast 45729.

Counsel and Care for the Elderly, 131 Middlesex Street, London E1 7JF.
01-621 1624.

Aims to give advice on any problem affecting an elderly person. Grants are available for people in genuine need.

Lion Clubs International,
4 The Drive, Hove, Sussex.

An international benevolent organisation. Local branches operate a wide variety of welfare schemes for the elderly and handicapped. Local address can be obtained from head office.

Help the Aged, 32 Dover Street, London W1.
01-499 0972.

Provides educative pamphlets and visual aids for those who are involved with elderly people. Largest fund raising and campaigning body in the UK. Working for the needs of the aged in Britain and the Third World.

ATTENDANCE ALLOWANCE

Attendance Allowance Unit, Department of Health and Social Security, Norcross, Blackpool, Lancashire FY5 3TA

An allowance for those who are severely disabled physically and mentally and need looking after at home. See leaflets NI205 and NI196, available from your local security office.

Coping with Aging Parents

BATHING

Disabled Living Foundation, 346 Kensington High Street, London W14 8NS. 01-602 2491.

DLF has a vast store of information and advice for the disabled, and runs an aid centre.

Occupational Therapists.

Social Services Departments will put you in touch with the nearest Occupational Therapist, who will advise about aids and bathing methods.

District Nurses.

District Nursing Service can be contacted through your GP. They will also give advice about bathing and carry out baths.

BOWELS

Colostomy Welfare Group, 38/39 Eccleston Square, London SW1V 1PD. 01-828 5175.

This group provides welfare service for patients with colostomy.

CANCER

National Society for Cancer Relief, Mrs Duthie, Graham Dyke Avenue, Bo'ness, West Lothian. Bo'ness 3899.

Provides grants for food, bedding, clothing, nursing services, convalescence, fares for visiting and other amenities.

Marie Curie Memorial Foundation, 124 Sloan Street, London SW1 8BP. 01-730 9157.

Provides advice and counselling for patients and their families.

Marie Curie Memorial Foundation, Marie Curie House, 21 Rutland Street, Edinburgh. 031-229 8332.

Provides nursing home accommodation for cancer sufferers and gives assistance with day and night nursing at home.

Cancer Care and Rehabilitation Society, Lodge Cottage, Church Lane, Tinsbury, Bath, Avon. 0761 70731. Mrs K. Palmer, 3 Blackie Road, Edinburgh EH6 7NA. 031-554 1798.

Aims to help fellow sufferers and their families. Visits, organises social activities and fund raising. Financial aid is given in emergencies.

Cancer Prevention Society, Mr G. Edward Rushworth, 102 Inveroran Drive, Bearsden, Glasgow G61 2AT. 041-942 6128.

An A.B.C. of Services

DEAFNESS

British Association of the Hard of Hearing, 6 St James Street, London WC1N 3DA. 01-405 5182.

Local self-help groups for those who have suffered hearing loss.

Hearing Aid Council, 40a Ludgate Hill, London EC4.

Advice and information on all types of hearing aid available.

Royal National Institute for the Deaf, 105 Gower Street, London WC1E 6AH. 01-387 8033.

RNID branches also exist in Scotland. National organisation to promote research, advice and information on all aspects of deafness.

Albion Deaf Association, 1 Old Belfast Road, Luton, Bedfordshire.

Scottish Association for the Deaf, Scottish Centre for the Education of the Deaf, Moray House, Edinburgh EH8 8AQ.

A voluntary organisation responsible for co-ordinating the work of all organisations working with the deaf in Scotland.

DEATH

Death Grants, Department of Health and Social Security local office.

See leaflet No. NI49. When you can't afford a funeral, the Local Authority is obliged to arrange one. In financial hardship, contact previous employer. They may be able to offer assistance.

Cruse, 126 Sheen Road, London W14.
01-940 4818.
Mrs M. Barnes, 21 Castle Street, Edinburgh EH2 4DN.
031-225 7100.

Voluntary organisation which offers help with emotional, practical and social problems following death of a relative. Also organises holidays and social outings.

Widows Association of Great Britain, 56 Gainsborough Road, Grindon, Sunderland, Tyne and Wear. 07834 2556 or 0632 853868.

These voluntary organisations aim to provide support to widows.

Widow Friends Society, Nasmith House, 175 Tower Bridge Road, London SE1.

Consumers Association, 4 Buckingham Street, London WC2. 01-839 1222.

Their booklet *What to do when Someone Dies* provides very useful information on all aspects of death.

DEMENTIA

Alzheimer's Disease Society, Bank Buildings, Fulham Broadway, London SW6 1EP.
01-381 3177.

Scottish Branch:
67 York Place, Edinburgh EH1
031-556 3062.

National organisation which provides information, advice and support to those caring for all dementia sufferers. Local addresses available from central office.

NB. Senile dementia used to be the term used for irreversible mental deterioration occurring after the age of 70, while Alzheimer's Disease referred to a similar pattern of deterioration occurring in middle age. Nowadays this distinction is felt to be less important since the underlying brain pathology seems to be the same, no matter at what age the deterioration begins.

Scottish Health Education Group, Woodburn House, Canaan Lane, Edinburgh.

SHEG publish a useful leaflet called *Forgetfulness and the Elderly.*

Age Concern Greater London, 154 Knatchbull Road, London SE5.

Leaflet, *Forgetfulness in Old Age* is very helpful.

Orientation Aids, Eddleston, Peebles. 0721 07213.

A variety of orientation aids are available. Write for catalogue.

DENTAL PROBLEMS

DHSS

Leaflets No. NH.54 (Guide to Dental Treatment under the NHS) and No. D.11 (Guide to claiming free dental treatment for those not on supplementary benefits) are helpful.

Local branches of WVRS, Age Concern or Council for Voluntary Services.

Contact these organisations to seek voluntary transport to surgeries and hospital appointments.

DEPRESSION

Depression Associated, Mrs J. Stephenson, 19 Merly Way, Wimborne Minster, Dorset BH21 1QN.
0202 883957.

Voluntary organisation whose aim is to break the stigma associated with, to provide help for and to foster research into the problems of depression. Send SAE for information.

An A.B.C. of Services

DISABILITY

Disability Alliance, 21 Star Street, London W2 1QB. 01-402 7026.

An information and advice group, publishes annual *Disability Rights Handbook.*

Disablement Income Group, Attlee House, Toynbee Hall, 28 Commercial Street, London E1. 01-247 2128/6877.

An advisory service dealing with welfare and benefits.

Disablement Income Group (Scotland), 152 Morrison Street, Edinburgh. 031-228 1666.

Disabled Christian Fellowship, Mrs J. Wiltshire, 50 Clan Road, Kingswood, Bristol. 0272-616141

A support group which links members through correspondence, exchange of cassettes and by phone. Tapes and cassettes on free loan.

Disabled Living Foundation, 346 Kensington High Street, London W8. 01-602 2491.

Provides information on all aspects of disability, rights, benefits and services.

Welsh Council for the Disabled, 1 Fox Crescent Road, Caerphilly, Mid Glamorgan. 02221-869224.

Provides information and advice.

Scottish Committee for Disability, 5 Shandwick Place, Edinburgh EH3. 031-229 8632.

Supplies information about various facilities for disabled people in Scotland. It has a clothing advisor, and provides literature about mobility aids.

Crossroads Care Attendant Scheme, 11 Whitehall Road, Rugby, Warwickshire. 0788 61536.
Scottish Branch: 24 George Square, Glasgow G2. 041-226 3793.

This scheme offers home relief and personal care service by trained staff for severely disabled people. Operates on an emergency and regular basis. Contact central office for local contact.

National Council for Carers and Elderly Dependants, 29 Chilworth Mews, London W2. 01-262 1451.

Offers support, advice and sitting service to those looking after a dependant.

British Red Cross Society, 9 Grosvenor Crescent, London SW1. 01-235 5454.

Branches, addresses and telephone numbers will be found in local directories. They supply commodes, bedpans and urinals, plus waterproof sheets. Booklets on how to look after someone who is bedridden.

Coping with Aging Parents

District Nursing Service

Contact your GP or direct.

Home Help Service.
Make referral direct to local Social
Work Department.

Home Helps will shop and carry out
domestic tasks in the home.

Wireless for the Bedridden Society,
20 Wimpole Street, London W1.

Organisation which can provide radio
and television sets to those who are
bedridden and cannot afford to
purchase.

Department of Health and Social
Security. (See your local directory for
telephone number).

Ask for information regarding
Supplementary Benefits, Special
Amounts. An extra allowance can be
given to people who require special
diets, have special laundry needs: i.e.
dealing with incontinence and special
heating needs: Ask for Leaflet SB.17.
Single payments for exceptional
needs may be given to people who
require lump-sum payments to
purchase household equipment, fuel,
or have fuel debts. See Leaflet SB.16.

DRIVING

General Practitioners

If an elderly person with some degree
of mental infirmity or dementia still
drives a car, his or her doctor should
be contacted. If the person suffers
from dementia, the GP should inform
the Driving and Vehicle Licence
Centre at Swansea of this fact, since
such individuals are significantly at
risk.

EYESIGHT

Leaflet NHS.6 sets out services and
provisions for the care of sight under
the NHS.

Contact your local Department of
Health and Social Security for
information.

National Listening Library,
49 Great Cumberland Place, London
W1.
01-723 5008

Provides a 'talking book' service.

HOLIDAYS

Disabled Living Foundation
(see under Disability).

Provides advice about holiday
accommodation for the elderly
disabled.

An A.B.C. of Services

Holidays for the Disabled,
Mr Jack Stacey, 12 Ryle Road,
Farnham, Surrey GU9 8RW.

Organises holidays for disabled people
of all ages, at home and abroad.

Holiday Care Service, 2 Old Bank
Chambers, Station Road, Horley,
Surrey.
74535.

Provides advice on holidays for
elderly and disabled people. Advises
on sources of financial help and relief
sources while carers have a break.

SAGA Holidays,
119 Sandgate Road, Folkstone, Kent
CT20 2BN.
Houses Advice, Centre for Policy on
Aging, Nuffield Lodge, Regents Park,
London NW1 4RS. 01-722 8871.

Special private organisation which
arranges holidays for retired people.

HOUSING

Rent and rates rebates.

For advice on obtaining rent or rate
relief, see your local Health Visitor or
Social Services Department.

Modifications to the home.

If there are structural problems, such
as dampness, noise or smells, contact
the local Environmental Health
Officers Department. They will also
supply details of grants to have
modifications made. If you require
built-in aids, contact the local Social
Services Department or the Citizens'
Advice Bureau who will give
information about local resources.

Moving house.

'Where to live after retirement',
published by the Consumers'
Association, provides useful
information about housing.

Moving in.

If you are considering having an
elderly infirm relative move in with
you, we strongly advise that you
consider first contacting a
professional, such as a social worker,
to discuss alternative arrangements
such as sheltered housing, or other
residential accommodation. An
objective eye can help you reach a
decision, and alert you to problems
you may not foresee.

Coping with Aging Parents

Houses Advice Centre for Policy on Aging, Nuffield Lodge, Regents Park, London NW1 4RS. 01-722 8871

An information guidance and support service for old people's residential homes.

Housing Associations

National Federation of Housing Associations, 32 Southampton Street, The Strand, London WC1.

Scottish Federation of Housing Associations, 42 York Place, Edinburgh EH1 3JD. 031-556 1435.

Both organisations can provide information on specialist housing associations including those for the handicapped and the elderly.

The Abbeyfield Society, 35a High Street, Potters Bar, Herts.

All these organisations provide residential home care for the elderly.

British Red Cross Society, 9 Grosvenor Crescent, London 1X 7EJ.

Church Army Sunset and Anchorage Homes, CSC House, North Circular Road, London NW10.

Civil Services Benevolent Fund, Watermead House, Sutton Court Road, Sutton, Surrey.

Distressed Gentlefolks' Aid Association, Vicarage Gate House, Kensington, London W8.

The Friends of the Elderly and Gentlefolks' Help, 42 Ebury Street, London SW1.

Jewish Welfare Board, 315-317 Ballards Lane, London WC2.

The Religious Society of Friends, Friends House, Euston Road, London NW1.

The Salvation Army Women's Social Service, 280 Marr Street, Hackney, London E8.

HYPOTHERMIA

Department of Health and Social Security.

Leaflet SB.16 'Help with Heating Costs' gives information to help obtain allowances for fuel bills, etc.

An A.B.C. of Services

Gas, Electricity and Solid Fuel Heating Centres.

All these centres have information and advice leaflets, dealing with such matters as heating systems, easy payment schemes, insulation, aids for disabled people—such as special tape for old people with a weak grip, free safety checks for elderly people living alone, etc.

The Spacecoat, Rawlings House, Rawlings Street, London SW3. 01-589 0551.

Suppliers of a housecoat which is made of special insulating material which will not catch fire, and which retains a high degree of heat.

Electric Blankets.

Extra low voltage electric blankets are now available which can be left on all night, and which will remain safe, even if the old person is incontinent. Enquire at Boots Chemists Ltd.

INCONTINENCE

Disabled Living Foundation
(see address in Disability section).

Incontinence Clinics.

Specialist Incontinence Clinics are opening in various parts of the country. Ask your GP for details and referral.

Incontinence Laundry Service.

This service is now available in many areas, supplying disposable pads, pants and laundry services for soiled linen. Contact GP or Health Visitor for details.

Pads, pants, toilet aids etc.

The British Red Cross Society (for address see under Housing) will loan bedpans, urinals, rubber sheets and commodes.

Urinary Conduit Association, 36 York Road, Denton, Manchester. 061-336 8818.

Gives advice about aids to prevent incontinence.

ISOLATION

Multiple Sclerosis Society, 71 Grey's Inn Road, London WC1X 8TR and 27 Castle Street, Edinburgh EH2. 031-225 3600.

Publishes a *Directory for the Disabled* which lists ideas for hobbies and activities which can help reduce isolation for the elderly and disabled.

Talking Newspapers Association of UK, Mrs Deaper, 48 Leigh Road, Eastleigh, Hants. 0703-641 244.

Organisation which provides cassette tapes of newspaper contents.

Age Concern (numerous local branches—see your telephone directory).

Local Age Concern officers will provide lists of activity clubs and luncheon clubs for the elderly.

Community Volunteer Action Groups (various local group addresses can be obtained from Age Concern or Citizens' Advice Bureaux).

Worth contacting to see if they can provide a volunteer to visit an elderly person who has difficulty getting out and would welcome company.

Social Services Day Centres (see local Social Services Departments).

WVRS may be of help in providing transport to visit Day Centres, or even friends and family if the elderly person has difficulties.

See also section on 'Pets.'

LEGAL ISSUES

Power of Attorney.

If an elderly person becomes too ill or disabled to manage their own affairs, a solicitor can prepare a Power of Attorney which gives a named relative or friend the right to conduct the affairs of that person on their behalf (with the old person's full knowledge).

Curator Bonis (Scotland) and Court of Protection Order (England and Wales).

When an old person has become completely incapable of managing their affairs, the solicitor can prepare a Curator Bonis or Court of Protection order. Advice on these matters can be obtained from the Citizens' Advice Bureaux, Legal Advice Centres, and law centres. Addresses of the legal aid offices can be obtained from the Citizens' Advice Bureaux, or by writing to the Legal Aid Headquarters, Chancery Lane, London WC2.

An A.B.C. of Services

Wills.

Advice on drawing up wills, and other issues, can be obtained from a solicitor, or from the Legal Aid Centre. If no will exists, then all property is held in trust for sale. Funeral and estate expenses, debts and any other liabilities will be paid, and the remainder will then go to those who are said to be beneficially entitled.

MENTAL ILLNESS

National Association for Mental Health (MIND), 22 Harley Street, London W1 2ED. 01-637 0741.

Scottish Association for Mental Health, 67 York Place, Edinburgh EH1 3JD. 031-556 3062.

Very often, elderly people are either unwilling or unable to seek help for psychological problems, but you should not hesitate to call in the doctor if you suspect that any change has taken place in the mental health of the elderly person you care for. These organisations will provide further help and advice.

PENSIONS

Supplementary Benefits. (Applications from local Post Offices and DHSS Offices).
See form SB.1 'Cash Help.'
(See also 'Your Rights for Pensions and Guide to all Benefits and Entitlements' published by Age Concern, price 55p. Available from major branches of W. H. Smith.)

If an elderly person's total income is insufficient to meet their needs, they are entitled to claim supplementary benefits. For all information on the rights and benefits of the elderly and their supporters, contact the Disability Alliance (for the address see Disability).

PETS

Sometimes elderly people worry about caring for their pets as they become less able to do for themselves. At the same time pets can be an enormous source of support, emotional uplift and also a motivating force to get some exercise. Local voluntary services or local branches of Age Concern will help an elderly person to look after a pet, if it becomes difficult. 'Sitters' can be found to take on the care if he or she goes into hospital, through local voluntary organisations.

Remember that cats and budgerigars require less care, and do not need the exercise that a dog does. If you feel your elderly relative is sometimes isolated and disabled, consider what a present a budgie might be.

Coping with Aging Parents

PILLS

Scottish Health Education Group, Woodburn House, Canaan Lane, Edinburgh EH10.

SHEG publish helpful literature—list on request.

Pharmaceutical Society of Great Britain, 1 Lambeth High Street, London SE1. 01-735 9141.

If you have any difficulty locally in the types of dispensers or bottles given to an elderly person, or the size of print on the label, first ask your local chemists if they can provide large type labels, clear instructions, easier opening bottles, etc.
Any further difficulties can be dealt with if you contact the Pharmaceutical Society.

Dosett Box Dispensers, Cow & Gate Ltd, Trowbridge, Wiltshire.

Ask your local chemist for advice on such things as Medi-dos or Dosett Box dispensers.

Medi-dos Dispensers, Pharmagen Ltd, Chapel Street, Runcorn, Cheshire.

PUBLIC TRANSPORT

DHSS Mobility Allowance.

For those physically and mentally disabled under the age of 65, who cannot use public transport, financial help is provided through the mobility allowance to use other means of transport. Transport may be provided by volunteers from these organisations: WRVS, British Red Cross, Age Concern. (See local telephone directory for addresses.)

Centre for the Policy on Aging, Nuffield Lodge, Regent's Park, London NW1 4RS. 01-722 8871.

Transport and the Elderly: Problems and Possible Action is a comprehensive review of the transport needs of the elderly and includes a series of practical recommended actions.

An A.B.C. of Services

RETIREMENT

Retired Executives Action, Clearing House, Victoria House, Southampton Row, London WC1B 4DH. 01-404 0904.

This society aims to link retired executives who have professional skills and experience, with voluntary bodies throughout the UK with a view to work on an expenses-only basis.

The Daily Telegraph Guide to Retirement, by David Loshak, £1.25.

Available from your local bookshop.

Scottish Retirement Council, 212 Bath Street, Glasgow G2. 041-332 9427.

Provides information and guidance for retirement.

Pre-Retirement Association, 19 Undine Street, London SW17. 01-767 3225.

Provides expert guidance in retirement planning. The organisation has a comprehensive information and advice service which is freely available to its members.

Pre-Retirement Choice Magazine, incorporating *Life Begins at 50*, Bedford Chambers, Covent Garden, London WC2. 01-876 8772.

Wakes Educational Programme, Temple House, 9 Upper Berkeley Street, London W1. 01. 01-402 5608/9.

Provides information about continuing education in retirement.

SPEECH PROBLEMS

Chest, Heart and Stroke Association, Tavistock House, Tavistock Square, London WC1H 9JE. 01-387 3012.

Has informative leaflets regarding speech problems following a stroke.

National Association of Laryngectomies Club, 4th Floor, Michael Sobell House, 30 Dorset Square, London NW1 6QL. 01-402 6007.

Speech problems can arise following a stroke, Alzheimer's Disease, or operations on the throat. Speech therapists from these organisations can give advice on how best to communicate with people who have impaired speech.

TEETH

Leaflets NHS.4, D.11, are available from the local DHSS. Those who receive supplementary pensions are entitled to free dental treatment.

Coping with Aging Parents

TELEPHONE

Financial assistance may be available from the Social Services Department. See the local telephone directory for the number.

Special telephones with flashing lights or large numerals are available. Ask the Social Services Department for details.

TERMINAL CARE

Care Unlimited,
Tonbridge, Kent.

Offers a service similar to the Hospice movement.
The local Hospice, if there is one, may provide a community nursing service, or alternatively admit the terminally ill patient into the Hospice to control pain and to die in dignity. Help is offered to families during terminal illness and in subsequent bereavement. Consult your GP for details.

Averil Knight,
St Christopher's Hospice, Lawrie Park Road, Sydenham, London SE26.
01-778 9252.

Provides and stores information about the hospice movement.

Cruse, 6 Lion Gate Gardens, Richmond, Surrey, and at
21 Castle Street, Edinburgh EH2 3DN.
031-225 7100.

Cruse is a voluntary organisation which offers help with practical, social and emotional problems following the death of a relative.

The Voluntary Euthanasia Society, 13 Prince of Wales Terrace, London W8 5PG.
01-937 7770, and 17 Hart Street, Edinburgh EH1 3RO.
031-556 4404.

A society supporting the right of the terminally ill to die with dignity and in comfort.

WANDERING

British Red Cross Society, St John's Ambulance. See telephone directory for local address.

An alarm system can be borrowed for a small fee. It operates like a baby alarm and alerts the family when someone is wandering in another room.

Care Call Unit, Seton Products Ltd, Turbiton House, Meddock Street, Oldham, Lancashire.

Provides a call-button system.

An A.B.C. of Services

Medic Alert Foundation, 9 Hanover Street, London W1R 9HF.

At a nominal charge, Medic Alert provides a bracelet or necklet which is engraved with the wearer's particular condition, name and address.

St John's SOS Talisman, PO Box 999, Kettering, Northants.

The SOS talisman is very similar to the Medic Alert.

N.B. If a relative suffering from dementia wanders away and cannot be found, alert the police *immediately*.

WHEELCHAIRS

British Red Cross Society, WRVS. See your local directory for the telephone number.

These organisations may give wheelchairs out on loan, alternatively contact your GP, health visitor, district nurse or occupational therapist for advice.

Motability, Boundary House, 91-93 Charter House Street, London EC1M 6BT. 01-253 1211.

A registered charity which helps disabled people in receipt of mobility allowance to obtain new cars on lease or hire purchase. Used cars and battery powered wheelchairs on hire purchase.

DIRECTORIES AND HANDBOOKS

Charities Digest, Family Welfare Association, 501-505 Kingland Road, London E8. 01-254 6251.

A catalogue of all voluntary organisations in the United Kingdom, published annually.

Directory for the Disabled, compiled by Ann Dannborough & Derek Kinnade. Published by Woodhead & Faulkner.

A handbook of information and opportunities for the disabled and handicapped.

Directory of National Voluntary Organisations in Scotland, 1982. Available from the Scottish Council of Social Service, 18/19 Claremont Crescent, Edinburgh EH7

Catalogue of voluntary organisations in Scotland.

Disability Rights Handbook, Disability Alliance, 21 Star Street, London W2 1QB. 01-402 7026.

This handbook is published annually to give information about benefits and rights for elderly and disabled people.

Coping with Aging Parents

Voluntary Organisations Directory,
National Council for Voluntary
Organisations, 26 Bedford Square,
London WC1B 3HG.

A directory of voluntary
organisations.

Residential Facilities in Scotland,
Scottish Council of Social Service,
18/19 Claremont Crescent, Edinburgh
EH7

A directory of residential facilities in
Scotland for the disabled and
handicapped.

3 Problems of Mobility

For many people old age brings on a reduction in personal mobility. It would be unrealistic to expect every 80-year-old to walk 15 miles a day, although some are able to do so and more. However, everyone should expect to be able to walk sufficiently well to shop, care for themselves and take part in leisure activities which are reasonable for their age unless their muscles or joints or their nervous system, which controls and co-ordinates movement, are impaired by illness. Old age alone is not a cause of severe immobility, although the illnesses which occur in old age can be if they are not diagnosed or treated. It is important to take action early to prevent reduced mobility and maintain health and well-being in old age. Preparation for a healthy old age begins in the early years of adulthood with an outgoing, interested approach to life; it can also be further helped by attending pre-retirement courses which will help people think of how they can constructively use their leisure time, for retirement often means a reduction in the number of social engagements and the possibly unexpected loss of friends, colleagues or relatives. The number of hobbies and leisure activities open to elderly people is increasing, especially activities designed for disabled people. In addition to hobbies, sporting opportunities are now being made more readily available. Many local authorities offer special concessions to pensioners who wish to swim, or learn to swim, play bowls, study yoga or take up any other form of exercise.

As well as providing companionship, pets, especially dogs, can have a tremendous value in providing a reason for getting out, improving confidence in walking and distracting the person's attention from him or herself.

Disabled elderly people often encounter problems when attempting to use public transport, and more often than not will not venture outside because it is too much effort getting on and off public transport. Why not enlist the help of a friend or relative to take the elderly person out for a change, or investigate the possibility of gaining help from a local voluntary organisation and have a volunteer take out your relative?

Causes of Immobility

Feet

Disorders of the feet affect many old people more commonly and can have just as dramatic effect on walking as more serious conditions. Typical problems are corns, bunions, ingrowing or overgrown toenails, ulcers and arthritis of the small joints of the foot and toes.

Some of the problems are often self induced and are the result of poorly fitting shoes and slippers; however, many elderly have difficulty in bending over to reach their feet and are unable to use scissors sufficiently well to cut their toenails. Ideally most elderly people should be seen by a chiropodist at least every six weeks or so, especially if they are diabetic or have bad circulation in their legs.

Joints

Rheumatoid arthritis, osteoarthritis and ankylosing spondylitis—a disease affecting the spine, are all conditions which produce a great deal of pain. In severe cases operations can be performed to replace or completely immobilise the joint, otherwise anti-inflammatory pain-relieving medications, short wave diathermy and gentle exercise given by the physiotherapist are the principal treatments available. The Disabled Living Foundation have very useful information about the aids available to help arthritic people at home. You will find the address in Chapter 2.

Muscle wasting and weakness in old people often accompany joint disorders which reduce mobility. Gentle exercise whether given by assistance or carried out independently is most important to prevent muscle shrinkage and joint contractures.

Mental Infirmity

The elderly person who becomes depressed and withdrawn may be unwilling to move about. He or she will tend to withdraw from activities and spend the time curled up in bed or in a chair. This inactivity may lead to muscle weakness, consequent unsteadiness and immobility. Loneliness, recent bereavement, or the onset of senile dementia may also be a cause of depression. If your relative should show signs of depression try to discover the cause by listening and

Problems of Mobility

understanding. It may be that your relative fears death or feels impotent and no longer able to lead an active, interesting life. If you can find a role for your relative or give him or her a purpose in life, it may be possible to reduce the depression and the inactivity associated with it. Even the housebound or those confined to bed may be able to carry out a service via a telephone, write a letter or do craft work. Severe forms of depression in the elderly may include an irrational belief that a part of the body is not functioning properly or has been invaded by cancer. These false beliefs may produce many other symptoms, such as pain, weakness and immobility; consequently the elderly person believes that he or she is very ill and must remain in bed.

One in ten of people over 65 will be diagnosed as suffering from dementia. There are still very few who understand the problems this presents to carers, especially as the sufferer generally looks so physically well. The mobility problems associated with dementia often arise from reduced muscle power, especially in strength of grip, which makes it harder to adjust to unsteadiness. Anxiety, speed and frustration will make the person more resistive, confused and less able to manage.

Other problems arising from dementia include impaired co-ordination, making dressing and manipulating sticks or zimmers a major effort. Occasionally the sense of balance is impaired in dementia, and walking becomes very unsteady.

Stroke

Sadly more and more elderly people are suffering strokes, a condition resulting from brain damage caused by an interrupted blood supply to the brain. Each half of the brain has an independent blood supply; therefore it is usual for only one half of the body to be weakened or paralysed.

The exact effect of a stroke depends on the part of the brain which is affected. Often it is the area responsible for the control and co-ordination of movement, including the muscles used in swallowing and speaking. It is common for people who have a stroke to lose the ability to identify the position of joints or limbs unless they can see where they are. Sometimes this is further complicated, because the victim's sight has also been affected.

As well as causing great difficulty dressing, walking or performing any other action, a stroke may have serious emotional and psychological effects. Even the ability to think may be affected which can lead to confusion and frustration. This may be characterised by mood changes and weeping. It is not surprising to find that the victim becomes angry and depressed by the loss of function and finds it difficult to adjust to a limited level of ability.

Exercises are most important and they should begin as soon as possible after the stroke has occurred. For instance, if the legs and feet are weak or paralysed move them, from the knee and ankle joints, backwards and forwards. As the legs become strong encourage the person to take short, supported steps. Similar exercises will be required for the arms. To assist with finger movements place a wad of cotton wool or an orange in the palm of the hand and encourage the person to squeeze and relax their fingers. Do not allow your relative to languish in bed. It is very easy to become despondent and give up, knowing that ability has been lost, especially if the speech has been affected. With firm encouragement and determination it may be possible to regain much lost functioning. Once your relative starts getting up, he should wear strong shoes and, as soon as he is able, his own clothes as this really is a good morale booster. Progress can be very slow and improvement can continue for up to two years. In some instances the doctor may refer your relative to a geriatric day hospital where physiotherapists, occupational therapists, speech therapists and nurses can give intensive treatment and exercise to aid recovery. The professionals are also able to make home visits, so if your relative is not attending a hospital, ask your doctor or health visitor to make a referral.

It is most important to return to a normal life as soon as possible and although certain handicaps will make that process difficult, the Chest, Heart and Stroke Association have produced a booklet entitled *Return to Mobility*, which provides useful information and encouragement.

Transient Ischaemic Attacks

These attacks occur when there is a temporary reduction of the blood supply to a small area of the brain. Occasionally this can happen when there is a sudden turning of the head. The symptoms vary according to the part of the brain affected, but generally there is weakness of the arms and legs, and there may be temporary loss of alertness, difficulty in speaking and loss of sight. The symptoms appear suddenly and only last for a short time, but they can lead to falls, unsteadiness of gait and dizziness. There is no specific treatment other than making sure the person does not come to harm. He may be aware of what has happened and feel strange and frightened by the experience.

Breathlessness

This symptom is quite common in the elderly and is caused by diseases of the heart and lungs, such as congestive heart failure, bronchitis, emphysema and pneumonia. During the acute phases of these illnesses the elderly person can be immobilised and bedridden. It is far better that the person is not confined to bed for long periods because many complications can arise and make their condition much worse. Encouragement and assistance to get out of bed, sit on a chair supported by pillows and then to carry out gentle exercise of the legs, will help to prevent stagnation of the blood supply. Gentle circulation of fresh air, although not a draught of air, will also aid easier breathing. It is important to recognise that restrictions in mobility associated with many chronic conditions like bronchitis are often as much psychological as the results of physiological incapacity. Smoking may well have precipitated and aggravated these conditions and therefore it would be wise to encourage the old person to cut down or give up completely.

Parkinson's Disease

This is a condition of the brain which primarily affects the control of movement. It seems to be caused by a loss of nerve cells in that part of the brain responsible for muscle control. The disease is characterised by trembling of the hands and head and stiffness of some or all of the muscles including those muscles which are used in speech. There may be general slowing in movements which causes a small stepping, shuffling walk. Treatment can only reduce the symptoms and to find the most appropriate treatment required, the doctor may refer your relative to the geriatrician, a doctor who specialises in the illnesses and treatment of the elderly. This could mean that your relative will be asked to attend a day hospital or an out-patient clinic for a while, until the right medication and dose has been found to control the symptoms. Levodopa (L Dopa) is now regarded as the most effective treatment of Parkinson's Disease. Unfortunately it has rather unpleasant side effects such as nausea, vomiting and low blood pressure. If these symptoms arise do consult the doctor since it is often possible to split the morning dose to reduce the rapid build-up of the drug in the morning which produces these unpleasant side effects. Parkinson symptoms can appear in elderly people who are taking one of the major tranquillising medications such as Largactil, Melleril or Haloperidol. If these symptoms do appear the doctor should be consulted. He will then either reduce the drug or introduce one of the anti-Parkinson medications to combat the symptoms.

The Parkinson's Disease Society (81 Queens Road, London SW19 8HR, 01-946 2500) aims to encourage and raise funds for research and to help sufferers and their relatives with the problems arising from Parkinson's Disease. Particularly useful are two booklets: *Parkinson's Disease, A Booklet for Patients and Their Families*, and *Parkinson's Disease—Day-to-Day*, a booklet for those who are affected.

Falls

Apart from falls due to external causes, such as tripping over a carpet, there are falls which have an internal cause and are commonly known as 'drop attacks'. Characteristically they come on as a surprise, there are no warning signs such as dizziness or loss of consciousness and once the old person is on the floor he is unable to get up again by his own efforts. It is thought that these attacks are caused by a sudden blockage of both cerebral arteries, as a result of kinking and/or arthritic changes in the neck, brought on by a sudden neck movement.

If these attacks do occur in your relative, firstly, make sure that the environment is safe and that the old person will do himself as little damage as possible, especially making sure the fire is guarded. Always inform the doctor who will want to give a full examination to exclude other possible causes. If the falls are occurring frequently he may prescribe the wearing of a neck collar which will prevent neck movements, thereby minimising the falls.

It is also worth while remembering that elderly people fall because of visual disturbances. Many old people who use bi-focal lenses misjudge distances, particularly when going downstairs, because they fail to allow for the distortion caused by their spectacles.

As a result of previous falls an old person may lose confidence in the ability to walk. This in turn produces more anxiety forcing the person to hang onto objects with the hands while attempting to move around. The unsteadiness and 'shaky legs' syndrome follows and more falls occur. The physiotherapist can give advice about exercises and walking aids which will give much needed support and encouragement towards achieving independence.

How to Help

Safety in the Home

Accidents are a major cause of illness and death in the elderly today, because of their delayed reactions to danger and their diminished perception of the environment. Accidents are also most likely to occur when the person is cross or tired, or hurrying, when there is an argument or when someone in the family is sick. At these times the elderly person is less alert to the possibility of an accident. While it is not so easy to make the environment safe outside the house, it is possible to reduce the risk of falling at home by first of all ensuring that you know the capabilities and limitations of your relative. An occupational therapist can give you a very good picture of what the person can do safely. If you do not have this resource, observe the person closely as he does various tasks. It might be an idea to have an emergency plan ready in case something does happen. Whom will you call if your relative is hurt? How will you get him or her out in case of a fire? Do you have easy access to first aid equipment or a telephone? One of the most important ways to avoid accidents is to change the environment to make it safer. Check through the house, garden and outside pathway regularly; by doing this thoughtfully you may find a pavement that is cracked or a carpet that is not tacked down securely. A neat house is safer than a cluttered one. There are fewer things to trip over or knock over, and hazards are more easily seen.

Coping with Aging Parents

Here is a safety check list developed by the Royal Society for the Prevention of Accidents, for you to discover weak safety points in your elderly relative's home. This will enable you to take a critical look at your relative's home for accident risks and forestall accidents by making sure the environment is safe.

Tick item(s) needing attention:

Gas

blocked flues ☐
blocked burners ☐
gas meter out of easy reach ☐
damaged, or rubber, tubing ☐
smell of leaking gas ☐
loose gas taps ☐

Electricity

'crackling' or hot plugs ☐
cracked plugs ☐
electric meter out of easy reach ☐
electric blanket unsafe ☐
electric switch in bathroom ☐
frayed flexes ☐
broken sockets ☐
points overloaded with adaptors ☐
no return switches on stairs ☐
vacuum cleaner unsafe ☐

House

slippery outside steps ☐
uneven paths or yard ☐
outside lavatory—no light ☐
uneven floors ☐
bath too high ☐
damaged walls ☐
no handrail on steps ☐
no outside light ☐
unsafe stair handrail ☐
window cords unsafe ☐
no bath grip rails
   or safety strips ☐
damaged ceilings ☐

Fire

unsafe oil heater ☐
cracked plugs ☐
unguarded coal fire ☐
no metal ash can ☐
smoking chimney ☐
unsafe paraffin can ☐
flammable clothing ☐
uses candles ☐

Furniture & Fittings

bed too high for easy access ☐
cupboard shelves too high
   for easy reaching ☐
cooker in unsafe place ☐
too little ventilation ☐
stiff taps ☐
leaking water taps ☐
insufficient heating
   causing undue cold ☐
mirror too near fire ☐
loose stair rods ☐
wringer unsafe ☐
armchair too low
   for comfort ☐
kitchen shelves too high
   for easy reaching ☐
   or too low ☐
too much trailing flex ☐
unsafe locks on
   cupboard doors ☐
carpets worn or torn ☐
torn stair coverings ☐
broken window panes ☐
use of wooden dustbins ☐

Problems of Mobility

Minimising the Effects of a Fall

While some old people will still fall even after all precautionary measures have been taken, it is possible to make other preparations should the old person be at risk.

Make sure the whole house is warm to prevent hypothermia should the person be immobilised on the floor.

Teach the old person to raise himself from the floor, get the help of a district nurse or physiotherapist, and while she is there ask for instructions on how you can lift correctly. Organise some kind of alarm system to alert the neighbours, either a knocking code or a whistle the elderly person can wear around his neck. Be sure to tell the neighbours about such arrangements.

Any permanently weakened limb or extremity, perhaps resulting from a stroke is more likely to break, because its reduced use and reduced weight bearing produce a thinning of the bone. It is therefore necessary to take special care to avoid falls and bangs on the affected side.

Recognising Fractures

Many elderly people are admitted to hospital for treatment of a fractured femur, because their bones become thinner with age and more susceptible to injury. This can be associated with a loss of calcium from the bones and a diet low in vitamin D. If you suspect that your relative has fractured his/her femur, contact the doctor. The signs and symptoms to look out for in a suspected fractured femur are:

Inability to get up after the fall, and to bear weight on one leg. Any movement of the hip causes severe pain.

Marked turning out of the leg and foot.

Shortening of the leg by approximately two-three centimetres.
Do not attempt to lift the person by yourself. Either wait for the doctor to arrive or call a neighbour, the police or the ambulance. In the meantime, keep the person warm, but do not give anything to eat or drink as he/she may require a general anaesthetic soon after being admitted to hospital.

Coping with Aging Parents

Care of the Immobilised Person at Home

Nursing your elderly relative at home means identifying the following possible problem areas and providing conditions that will enable him, unaided, to gain independence as quickly as possible.

Problem	*Action*
Breathing	Use a back rest or plenty of cushions or pillows to help the person breathe more comfortably. Make sure he takes prescribed medication regularly. Have a gentle circulation of fresh air in the room, but avoid draughts.
Eating and Drinking	Offer frequent small attractive snacks. Eat with your relative. Try Complan or Carnation Breakfast to supplement diet if full diet is refused. Have drinks available and accessible in a non-spill cup.
Going to the Toilet	Provide easy access to toilet, commode or urinal. To prevent incontinence, remind person to use the toilet every two hours. Borrow or hire aids if necessary. Provide receptacle or tissues for disposal of chest phlegm.
Washing	Regular bath or wash down in bed. Bath aids are available. Enlist help of district nurse if necessary.
Dangers in the Environment	Regular house checks for poorly laid carpets, lino etc. See list on previous page.
Sleep	Try to keep the person awake and active through the day by providing stimulation. Make sure the bed is warm and comfortable, and that the person is pain free and not suffering from pressure sores, and visits the toilet prior to retiring. Warm, milky drink can be given to aid sleep. Make sure he/she feels safe in the environment.

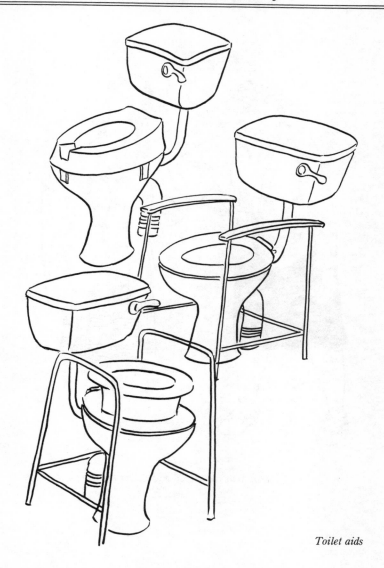

Toilet aids

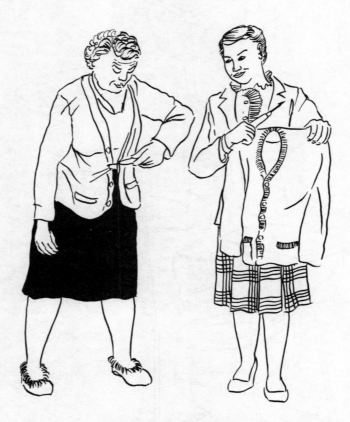

Help your relative to dress rather than doing it for her

Problems of Mobility

Dressing

Allow plenty of time to get ready, lay out the clothes in the order in which they are to be worn and then instruct the person to fit the garment over the weak part of the body first. To make fitting easier, zip and button fastenings can be replaced by Velcro tape; various dressing aids can also be obtained from the occupational therapist to make the task easier.

Keeping Warm

Make sure there are sufficient finances to cover the cost of heating by checking the benefits that are available. Electric bed blankets are now available with inbuilt safety precautions. Have them checked from time to time. An adequate diet maintains internal warmth and energy. Thermal underwear is a good conserver of heat. Encourage gentle exercise to avoid poor circulation.

Communication

Listen, have patience, do not take over. Work with your relative. Encourage communication with others. Invite friends, neighbours and relatives to the house. Act as your relative's advocate.

Gaining Independence

Break down the tasks into achievable aims. Have low expectations, slowly build upon your relative's achievements. Give encouragement and let the person know how they are doing. Do not assume your relative knows you are pleased with his progress.

Recreation

Encourage young people to visit, ask them to take part in chess games, cards, discussion of books or whatever may interest your relative. Maybe visitors will take your relative out, in a wheelchair or to have a short walk.

Once you have enlisted all the help you can in the form of aids, services and people, be sure to encourage your relative to do as much as possible, no matter how simple or difficult the task may be.

Preventing Pressure Sores

Unless the elderly person is acutely ill it is not advisable to have him stay in bed for long periods. This can produce serious chest, circulatory and urinary tract complications and prolong the period of immobility unnecessarily. For those who are immobile and spend long periods in bed or sitting in a chair, there is a risk of developing a pressure sore. These are wounds caused by constant pressure of a bed or chair on any part of the body causing a diminished blood supply. Any elderly person who is: over sedated and drowsy, undernourished, anaemic, incontinent, deteriorated mentally or inactive is at risk of developing pressure sores.

To prevent their development the person must be given a well-balanced diet with plenty of fluids. He should be systematically turned at least every two hours from the left side to the right. Gentle massage of the reddened areas with talcum powder or a light cream will help to restore the blood supply to the affected area. If the person is incontinent, the bed and nightclothes should be changed regularly and the wet area washed and dried thoroughly. A light application of zinc and castor oil ointment can be made to replace the natural oils lost through frequent washing. Do not forget to change the sitting position should your relative be spending long periods in the chair. An inflatable or foam rubber ring will help to relieve the pressure.

The Red Cross lends such aids as bed pans, commodes and back rests to people who are being nursed at home, but it would be best to consult the district nurse who can advise about the availability of such aids. Marino sheepskins are most comfortable to lie on and do help in the prevention of bed sores, but they are of little use if your relative is incontinent. They also tend to be rather expensive.

Help with Washing and Bathing Difficulties

Washing and bathing pose difficulties for some elderly people. The main problems encountered are those due to loss of power in one hand or arm, limitations of shoulder and hip movements, disturbance of

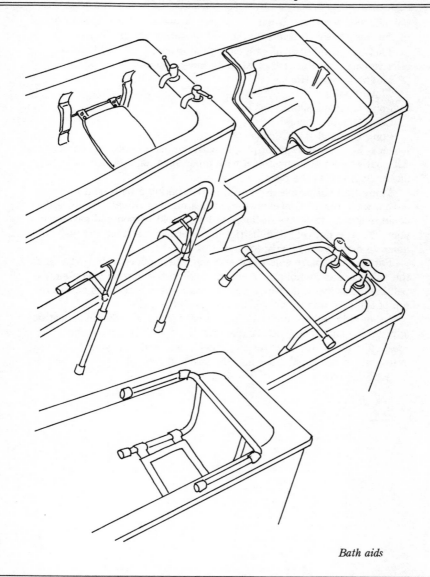

Bath aids

balance and dementia. It may be useful to suggest that sitting in front of the wash basin to complete the task in safety will be easier.

There are a number of gadgets on the market that will help your relative carry out the task of washing independently:

Magnetic Soap Holder
Glove Sponge
Long Handled Sponge
Long Handled Loofah
Long Handled Back Brush

Roller towels are easiest for people with the use of only one hand. Alternatively an ordinary towel with tapes sewn on and tied to hooks on the wall serves the purpose.

Many frail old people are afraid to risk taking a bath, and prefer to have a wash down. However, there are a number of aids available that could make the task less frightening for the old person and easier for yourself. Alternatively, the district nurse or her assistant will visit the home to bathe your elderly relative.

For those who are able to sit and stand unsupported, but who lack the balance and confidence to enter a bath in the normal way a simple bathing aid is available which consists of a board which lies across the top of the bath and a seat which sits inside the bath.

Other aids include various types of bath seats, a bath safety mat and adjustable hand rails. The occupational therapist can advise about the most suitable aid for your relative's need, and will visit your home to assess his or her capabilities and the size and type of bathroom before prescribing aids.

4 Failing Senses

In order to manage our everyday life, we must communicate with the world. Our senses provide us with our principal means of staying 'in touch'. Although sight and hearing are the most obvious senses through which we know what is going on around us, smell, taste and touch are equally important to our appreciation of the world. With increasing age there may be some decline in our sense of smell, taste and touch, but only very rarely is there complete failure of any of these senses. In contrast, deafness and blindness affect a significant minority of older people, while reductions in hearing and vision which interfere with the normal activities of daily life are common.

One unfortunate consequence of the view that old age and infirmity are one and the same, is the small number of elderly people who bother to get regular checks of their sight and hearing. Before considering specific problems associated with difficulties in seeing and hearing, it is important to stress the value of regular check-ups, even if there are no obvious complaints or signs of deafness or loss of vision. Many conditions develop silently and slowly and detection is made too late. Encouraging the elderly to have their eyes and ears checked costs nothing—and can be of great benefit.

Vision

One of the commonest causes of failing vision in the elderly is *cataract*: a thickening of the lens or part of the lens which causes dimming of vision, afterwards accompanied by a pinkish colouring of sight. Depending upon the type and stage of the process, treatment may involve eyedrops, new glasses, or an operation.

A second group of less treatable conditions are those responsible for producing damage to the retina (the screen of tiny nerve endings at the back of the eye). They may be the result of illness primarily affecting other organs, such as diabetes or high blood pressure, or (less often) a localised destruction of the blood supply to the retina. The result is 'blind spots' of varying degree, which interfere with vision, rather than total blindness.

Glaucoma, the name given for raised pressure of the fluid within the eye, usually begins after the age of fifty. It can have a sudden onset of pain and blurred vision, or take a slowly progressive course, which may not be noticed early on. There is a gradual dimming of vision, particularly for the areas *surrounding* the central focus of sight, while the centre of vision is unaffected. One common effect is that sources of light seem to be surrounded by a kind of halo.

Early recognition is important so that treatment can be instituted to prevent any progressive deterioration. Treatment is usually with eyedrops, often supplemented by tablets. The medicine-taking regime can be extremely complicated and confusing to an elderly person—one lady had four different eyedrop bottles, and four different bottles of tablets to take, each at differing times. The instructions (when and how many drops) were written only on the boxes (which she discarded) and not on the bottles themselves. Advice on dealing with these sorts of problems is given in the chapter on Medicines.

While not affecting the eye itself, *strokes* can damage centres in the brain responsible for the experience of seeing, causing visual field defects (blind regions within the area of vision). The effects can vary, but include such problems as apparent blindness in one eye, as though half of the vision were blacked out. There is often a gradual recovery process after the stroke.

Soreness and reddening of the eyes can be another common problem for elderly people, often associated with a condition called *ectropion*, when the muscles in the eyelids weaken, making them fold back and become less efficient in cleaning and wiping the eyeball. Sometimes the reverse happens, and the eyelids turn inwards (*entropion*) producing considerable soreness.

Leaflet NHS6 sets out the services and provisions available under the National Health Service for the care of sight. Examinations can be made without charge by an ophthalmic medical practitioner or an ophthalmic optician. Additional advice on such aids as magnifying glasses or special spectacles for those confined to bed can be obtained from the Disabled Living Foundation or the Disability Alliance (for addresses see Chapter 2).

For elderly people partly or totally blind, it is important to attend to safety factors in the home. Seek advice on any modifications that can be made—such as installing a handrail to help guide the person from the bedroom to the bathroom—by contacting your local social services department. Dangerous features about the house can be checked through the checklist on home safety provided by the Royal Society for the Prevention of Accidents (see Chapter 3).

Failing Senses

Many libraries offer a 'talking book' service which can be a great boon to people who can no longer enjoy normal reading. Special allowances are available for the purchase of radios, another means of reducing isolation. The Royal National Institute for the Blind also have their own talking book services, as well as much useful information for both the blind and their relatives regarding ways of reducing the disabilities associated with blindness. Their address is given in Chapter 2.

It is important to help reduce the isolation that can accompany any such disability. Because letters cannot be read, ask friends and relatives to make tape cassettes to pass on news and greetings. By helping an elderly person to get used to handling a cassette player, you can open up opportunities which will go some way to compensating for the losses associated with blindness. The 'speaking clock' on the telephone can provide a ready means to check on the time, as an alternative to the radio.

Hearing

Although deafness is a disability in some ways similar to the loss of sight, it has effects on everyday social life which are not evident in the case of the partly sighted or blind. When we converse with a blind person, touch and tone of voice do much to convey our physical presence and personal concern in a subtle way that words alone cannot do. Talking with someone who is deaf or hard of hearing is all too often like a continual quarrel!

The deaf person often talks loudly without realising it, while the other also shouts to make himself heard. Misunderstandings and missed messages do much to add to the frustration on both sides. In this way, the quality of human contact seems to be more affected by hearing loss than the loss or partial loss of sight.

While obvious deafness is easily recognised and acted upon, many elderly people suffer from losses of hearing clarity which can only be detected through careful clinical examination. Such mild losses can have serious implications in terms of increasing confusion, activating suspicion and increasing social withdrawal. There is sometimes a progressive loss of hearing, affecting both ears equally, especially noticeable with higher frequencies, and making the discrimination of sounds more difficult, rather than the hearing of the sound itself—'th's'

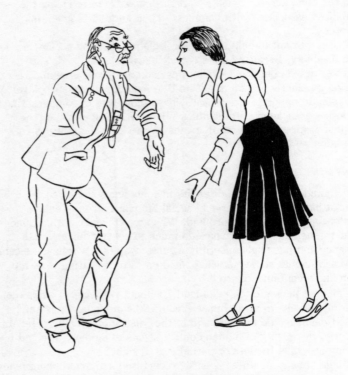

Talking with a deaf person can seem like a continual argument

Failing Senses

confused with 'f's', 'sh's' with 's's', etc. The basis for this loss is a deterioration in the nerves responsible for conducting sounds from the ear to the brain, and while various aids can help compensate for the hearing loss, there is little likelihood of reversing the process. Fairly sudden hearing loss is relatively rare and always requires investigation. *Tinnitus*, the hearing of noises in the head or ears, described as hissing, ringing or rushing sounds, can be extremely distressing and disturbing, and reassurance and advice from a doctor can be helpful. A final problem that can be overlooked is simply the build-up of wax in the ears—a very curable source of hearing difficulties!

Help for the hard of hearing can obviously come from the doctor—regular checkups are always important. He can refer the patient to the local Hearing Aid Distribution Centre. Advice and information on hearing aids can be obtained from the Royal National Institute for the Deaf, who will also suggest ways and means of improving communication generally—such as details of special door bell systems and telephones. The British Association of the Hard of Hearing is another organisation that produces leaflets and information of value to the partially deaf. Addresses for both these organisations are in Chapter 2.

All the purely technical aids require regular servicing and checkups. You should make sure that, if an elderly person has stopped using an aid because 'it's no good', the fault does not lie in faulty working—or indeed in a buildup of wax in the ear caused by the insertion of the ear-piece. This latter problem is not uncommon, and all hearing-aid users should have regular inspections of their ears to make sure they are free of wax.

On a more day-to-day level, there are certain guidelines that can be useful when communicating with the hard of hearing. First, *don't shout*. A very loud voice is not a very clear voice— shouting just adds to confusion and anxiety. Secondly, speak slowly and clearly and don't hide your mouth. Letting the person see you speaking increases the cues that can help him comprehend what you are saying. Pausing between phrases and sentences helps reduce problems of 'blurring' and makes speech more distinct. Lowering the tone of your voice may also be helpful to some people with hearing loss. Thirdly, if the person uses a hearing aid, make sure you know how it works, how it should be fitted, and how to adjust it. If the person is inclined to get confused or is forgetful, remember to check batteries and see that the device is properly fitted in the ear, gets taken out and switched off at night-time and so on. Fourthly, check that what you are saying is understood.

Deafness can make some elderly people touchy and suspicious of others. If you know the person has always been rather touchy and distrustful, it is especially important to avoid misunderstandings. In situations where a number of people are talking, be prepared to sit next to the person and help him keep up with what is being said. Don't encourage the person to give up on social intercourse just because it's difficult to follow, and take part in, general conversation.

Summary

1: Regular checkups of sight and hearing for all over-65s are highly desirable, whether or not you are having difficulties.

2: Sudden changes in hearing or sight are very rare, and almost always important—do see your doctor in such circumstances.

3: For those with partial losses—of sight or hearing—aids such as spectacles, magnifying glasses, hearing aids, communicators, need regular checks as well. No aids are perfect, but faulty aids can be worse than useless.

4: For those with major impairment of sight, get expert advice on safety factors in the home (ROSPA), talking books (Library Service, RNIB), and try to encourage the use of a cassette player, both for entertainment (you can make up your own book service!), passing on news and greetings from relatives who cannot visit regularly, and as a local 'talking newspaper'.

5: For those with major impairment of hearing, get help and advice from the BAHH and RNID.

Note: For addresses see Chapter 2.

Problems Associated with Brain Damage

Communication problems can also arise from damage to those centres inside the brain responsible for interpreting and understanding incoming information from the eyes and ears. Strokes and degenerative diseases of the central nervous system can interfere with our perception of the world, so that language or the nature and use of

The message inside this card reads

Lots of Happiness
for the future.

Have a Wonderful Retirement.

REGAL GREETING CARDS LTD.

Failing Senses

objects are not correctly understood. The words are heard, but convey no meaning (*aphasia*), or objects are seen, but there is no understanding of what they are (*agnosia*).

These disabilities are often missed, and the elderly individual is seen simply as 'confused' or 'muddled'. Professional evaluation—by a neurologist, or speech therapist—is important, so that he can test whether these disabilities are present. If you suspect that sometimes the elderly person you care for cannot make sense of what is said, or seems to be puzzled by everyday objects, contact your doctor and ask him to refer the matter to a specialist.

At a practical level, short straightforward questions and statements with only one 'message' will be least taxing to grasp for someone with aphasia. Going on and on, speaking quickly, asking several questions at once will only confuse. For someone with agnosia (not recognising objects) it is harder to compensate for such disabilities, and the condition is often difficult to distinguish from general confusion. Professional advice from a specialist is needed here, so ask your doctor about referral to a specialist.

Finally, if speech is affected by a stroke or other neurological disorder (*expressive dysphasia*), it is helpful to receive guidance from a qualified speech therapist. The problem may be a difficulty in articulation, rather than in the ability to express meaning, or may involve both. Often stress and frustration make such difficulties much worse, and it is important to avoid prolonged attempts to understand which are leading only to upset. Supplying the word, if it cannot be found, asking the person to point or gesture, checking wrong use of words and supplying the correct one all can help if done with patience, a sense of humour and a readiness to stop and try again later.

5 Problems with Diet

Nutrition is one of the factors which determine how long we live. A good diet will help us to live out our full lifespan, while a poor diet will shorten life. There are very few fat people over 80 simply because fat people generally don't live to a great age.

The nutritional needs of old people are exactly the same as for any other group, but the quantity required may be a little less due to the reduced amount of physical energy expended. What is important is taking various sorts of nourishment in the right proportions and quantities. A well-balanced diet should include meat, fish, vegetables, bread, milk and fruit, and most importantly fibre, which is contained in wholemeal bread, fresh fruit, vegetables and bran. Fibre is the substance which produces bulk in the stool and if taken regularly it will prevent constipation.

For the majority of elderly people living in Britain, obtaining enough to eat is not a problem, but some old people do not get enough of the right foods.

Incorrect nutrition may show itself either as under-nutrition or as obesity. Either of these may lead to disease; for instance, during the winter months many elderly people are admitted to hospital suffering from bronchitis or pneumonia, which may be a consequence of a poor diet leading to lowered resistance to infection.

Much attention these days is also given to the relationship between the intake of animal fats and hardening of the arteries, which can result in angina, heart attacks and strokes.

Identifying Those at Risk

Eating is a complex physical, psychological, social and cultural activity; it is perhaps not surprising, therefore, to find that there are many factors which may affect the intake of food and the nutritional status of an elderly person.

This chapter aims to identify those elderly people at risk of having an inadequate diet, some common problems which may arise as a result, and ways in which the problems can be tackled.

Mealtimes are generally regarded as pleasant social landmarks in the day, and most people tend to make them a central part of their lives. However, as people reach old age there may not be the same social opportunities either to prepare a meal for guests or to be invited

Problems with Diet

out, and when social life is diminishing, the pleasures of eating seem to evaporate too. Loneliness is probably one of the biggest appetite suppressants there is.

The elderly, especially the recently bereaved or those who live alone, may feel that they have little incentive to prepare food for themselves. This reluctance to prepare food may be further complicated by a diminished sense of taste and smell, in addition to a less active stomach. Widowed men are particularly at risk since they may have relied totally on their wives to prepare meals. They may be inexperienced in domestic matters, spending money unwillingly or unwisely—for example, on alcohol rather than on solid food. Over-indulgence in alcohol in elderly people is not uncommon; it may be skilfully hidden and is often an indication of an underlying depression resulting from loneliness.

Impaired mobility could result from such conditions as Parkinson's Disease, arthritis, stroke and chronic chest problems, and may make elderly people reluctant to go shopping; this can be further aggravated by a low income and the ever-increasing price of food.

Generally speaking, the digestive system of an elderly person is perfectly healthy and the ability to absorb food and liquid is not impaired, but the presence of untreated dental decay or ill-fitting dentures may prevent the intake of regular meals. Loss of teeth, pain or poorly fitting dentures can reduce the ability to chew properly, and if the enjoyment of food is lost through discomfort then it is not surprising if people eat less.

Difficulty in swallowing obviously impairs the intake of food, and may be due to a number of causes: most frequently in the elderly it follows a stroke, because damage has occurred in the area of the brain that is responsible for the swallowing action. This difficulty is usually temporary, and it may be necessary to follow very careful feeding instructions given by the doctor until swallowing has returned.

Hiatus hernia, a protrusion of part of the stomach into the chest region, is another relatively common complaint which can impair food intake; it causes considerable pain and discomfort and requires prompt medical care. Stomach and bowel operations, whether recent or long past, may also be a factor. If stomach and bowel disorders persist and the elderly person won't eat properly, consult the doctor; but also make sure your relative is sticking to any specially prescribed diet.

Mental Disturbances

Many elderly people experience emotional disturbances which affect their ability to eat properly. Depression is one such condition; it occasionally occurs for the first time in old age, but it is more usual to find that it appeared in earlier life and continued or recurred in old age. In more severe cases of depression, marked loss of appetite and weight loss are apparent; the situation may be further complicated by the presence of delusions such as 'My bowels are blocked and I cannot eat' or 'I have no money to buy food'. Occasionally the person may have paranoid ideas and thinks, for example, that the food is poisoned. These symptoms usually appear gradually; in the early stages it may be possible to distract the person from the symptoms and then encourage his eating. It may not be so easy in the acute phase, when the person is adamant about refusing food. The best solution is not to go on fighting but call the doctor, who in turn may request an assessment by the psychiatrist.

Forgetful people, those who are suffering from dementia, and especially those who live alone, may forget to eat even if food is left out. They may hide food, throw it away or eat it after it has spoiled. These are signs that the person can no longer manage alone, and that new arrangements must be made. You can possibly manage for a time by telephoning at meal times to remind your relative to eat, or you may be able to set an alarm clock beside a flask of soup and some sandwiches. People with dementia may be unable to recognise that some things are not good to eat, or sometimes they may forget that they have already taken a meal, and want to eat again. Try putting out a plate of small snacks, such as biscuits and cheese, or pieces of apple and celery. It may be very difficult to institute a foolproof method of ensuring that your relative eats regularly and in some instances the only solution is to have someone sit down and take a meal with your relative.

If the dementia sufferer has problems with co-ordination he or she may lose the ability to feed properly. Use a plastic tablecloth or plastic placemat, and get the person a plastic apron to wear. Try putting out only one utensil (a spoon is probably the most useful); cut the food into small manageable pieces, and serve it in a bowl which is a different colour from the tablecloth. It may also be easier if the bowl is placed on a non-slip surface, such as a damp cloth. To keep food from being pushed off the plate, use a plate guard. Domiciliary occupational therapists will give advice about helpful aids to use at meal times and can be contacted at the social services department.

Someone with dementia may lose the ability to judge how much liquid will fill a glass. He or she will need your help to pour, especially when serving hot liquids; do not fill glasses or cups right to the top, and if necessary use a cup with a spout to prevent spills. Be sure that the person gets enough fluid each day; memory-impaired people can forget to drink. Limit the number of foods you serve; for example put out only one food at a time, such as a small portion of meat followed by vegetable; this may make eating easier. Do not leave condiments on the table where they can be reached and mixed into the food inappropriately.

If your relative requires spoon-feeding, put only a small amount of food on the spoon at a time, and wait until the food is swallowed before offering more. You may have to remind him or her to swallow, or help by gently stroking the throat.

Dietary Problems

Obesity

Overweight people are prone to many diseases, and many conditions can be made worse by overweight—for instance diabetes, high blood pressure and chronic chest problems. An obese person will recover more slowly from illness even if the illness is unconnected with the overweight.

The commonest cause of obesity is straightforward—more food is consumed than is required for a day's work, and the surplus is converted to fat. However, before embarking on a diet it is worth while checking with the doctor, as some illnesses cause people to gain weight. Seek help from the health visitor or dietician who will suggest the most suitable diet. Otherwise it is worth encouraging your relative to reduce the intake of fats and sugar and to increase the intake of fibre. Encourage the old person to take exercise; having a pet (if living at home) may provide a distraction from eating and a stimulus to take exercise.

Coping with Aging Parents

Constipation

One of the commonest ailments of old age is constipation, a condition which can be remedied relatively easily, but which can produce a variety of physical problems and even mental confusion.

Constipation is characterised by the difficult passage of hard stools; in extreme cases it can produce diarrhoea, when the very hard faeces in the large bowel cause an irritation to the lining, which in turn produces an excessive amount of mucus which leaks past the hard mass. There are five main causes of constipation.

1: Inadequate intake of fibre and liquid in the diet, which may be the result of life-long habits including the taking of laxatives.

2: Reduced peristaltic action (the digestive tract movement to push foods through the stomach and bowel) due to disease.

3: Reduced mobility and exercise due to physical infirmity or depression. The bedridden are particularly prone to constipation.

4: Dementia sufferers cannot remember to empty their bowels, or they cannot identify the signal to do so.

5: Side-effects from medicine, particularly those containing codeine.

Many elderly people are obsessed with their bowel actions and in order to have a daily movement will purge themselves with a variety of laxatives. This routine has probably lasted a long time, and for some no amount of education and retraining will change their routine, because their mind and body has been conditioned to function only with the use of a laxative.

To prevent or correct constipation you should advise your relative to take a diet containing plenty of fibre, such as wholemeal bread, bran, vegetables, fresh fruit and liquid. Regular gentle exercise will also help. For some the diet and exercise alone will not remedy the constipation, but before allowing your relative to take any type of laxative do consult the doctor, who will advise on the most appropriate ones. In severe cases of constipation the doctor may recommend the insertion of suppositories or an enema; however, if this is prescribed, the district nurse will usually be asked to call to carry out the procedure. It may also be useful for the doctor to give your relative a complete physical examination to make sure the constipation is not connected with any other illness.

Problems with Diet

Piles

Constipation invariably aggravates piles or haemorrhoids, a painful, irritating condition resulting from dilated veins in the rectum. The common symptoms are pain, discomfort and bleeding. If the person passes blood or black motions, consult the doctor, especially if the bleeding is heavy or persistent. Although haemorrhoids may be the cause, it is important to exclude other more serious causes.

There are many over-the-counter remedies for piles, but it is far better to be guided by the advice from the doctor. Prevention of constipation and general skin care are just as important as the treatment of piles. If your elderly relative is mobile, a daily lukewarm bath is most comforting, but special care should be taken to dry the genital and anal area. If he or she is bedridden, a twice-daily wash down will do just as well. The surgical removal of piles is a most painful operation and is only recommended if there is persistent bleeding, which may lead to anaemia, or if there is a lot of pain.

Diarrhoea

As previously mentioned, diarrhoea can be the result of severe constipation, where hard stools in the lower end of the bowel irritate the sensitive lining of the bowel, causing it to produce mucus, which leaks out of the back passage and gives the appearance of diarrhoea on the person's underwear and bedclothes.

Other causes include:

1: Food poisoning which produces sudden watery stools and may be accompanied by vomiting.

2: Diverticulitis (an inflammation of the bowel lining) may produce alternate constipation and diarrhoea.

3: Some drugs may produce diarrhoea as a side effect.

If diarrhoea lasts for more than two days, consult the doctor; otherwise make sure your relative can reach the toilet in time, or has easy access to a commode. Giving plenty of fluid and keeping off solid food for a short while may help to give the bowel a rest.

Coping with Aging Parents

Indigestion

Indigestion or dyspepsia is another dietary problem which can worry and cause discomfort to elderly people. It is not a disease, but a symptom of an underlying condition. It is rarely serious, but if it persists and is very painful it could indicate the presence of an ulcer or hiatus hernia.

Indigestion is caused by too much hydrochloric acid in the stomach, a condition which can be aggravated by taking meals too quickly, insufficient chewing of food, or taking of indigestible foods or alcohol, tea, coffee, tobacco or some drugs. In addition, nervous tension or anxiety frequently causes gastric upset; most people have experienced loss of appetite, vague discomfort in the stomach, a feeling of nausea and similar symptoms when they are under some strain.

There are a variety of medicines available to allay the symptoms of indigestion; a suitable one may be recommended by the chemist. If the discomfort persists it could lead to the person eating less and losing weight. Do consult the doctor rather than try to treat your relative yourself.

Weight Loss

Sometimes a person with or without dementia loses weight; this may be related to a refusal to take food, and it may come on gradually. It could signal the presence of a physical disorder. Check whether the person is depressed, has an acute illness, or has had a stroke. Be sure to search carefully for any other contributing factor. If there is a marked loss of weight over a period of time, consult the doctor.

Diabetes

Mild diabetes is common in the elderly. It may go undetected for a number of years, and only be discovered after a routine blood or urine test. Symptoms can include frequent passing of urine, even during the night, thirst, and sometimes a change of bowel habit and weight loss. It is most important that the diabetic patient is thoroughly assessed as an individual. There are now many diabetic clinics functioning as part of the out-patient department of the general hospital; be sure to ask about this facility if your elderly relative is diagnosed as having diabetes.

Problems with Diet

The British Diabetic Association, 10 Queen Ann Street, London W1M 0BD (tel. 01-323 1531) is careful to refer queries to the diabetic's own doctor if possible, but free advice is given on diet, employment, education, insurance and travel. It produces a newsletter six times a year.

Approaches to Diet Problems

If you know that your relative is at risk of not eating properly, there are certain steps which you can take. The problem is not easy to spot. If your relative is losing weight it can be easier to identify, but a person can develop malnutrition without obvious weight loss. Other signs to watch for are a painful tongue and sores at the corners of the mouth.

Shopping

First, make sure that your relative is receiving all the financial benefits for which he is eligible. Secondly, sit down with him or her to plan a weekly food budget, bearing in mind that daily consumption should include at least half a pint of milk, some fruit for vitamin C, a portion of fish, meat, poultry, cheese or eggs, and some wholemeal bread or breakfast cereal rich in natural fibre. Whenever possible encourage elderly people to shop for their own needs or to accompany someone else; the exercise will do them good. For some the journey to the shops is far too tiring or too much to cope with; the alternative is to ask local shopkeepers to deliver to the home. A helpful neighbour or the Home Help could do the shopping; whoever is going to be responsible, do encourage the helper to include the elderly person in some part of the task.

It is wise to have an emergency store of food which can be topped up with items bought at the end of the week, if there is money left over. In times of bad weather or illness, it may not be possible to get to the shops.

Suggested contents for Emergency Stores Cupboard:

Complan or similar products.	Fruit juice.
Breakfast cereal.	Soup: tins, packets.
Milk: tinned, dried, long-life.	Main course: tinned fish or meat.
Biscuits: sweet, plain.	Vegetables: dried or tinned.
Drinks: tea, coffee, cocoa, beefy preparations.	Potatoes: tinned or instant, with Vitamin C added.

Coping with Aging Parents

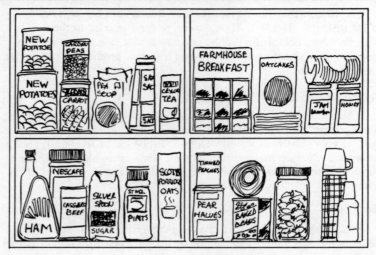

A well-ordered emergency store cupboard

A refrigerator, and cupboards which are easily accessible, are the ideal places to store food. Regular checks on the contents will keep you informed as to the old person's food intake; a surreptitious look into the waste bin will also give you a clue to the eating habits of your relative. It is important to note the expiring date on the cans or packets of food.

Catering for One

Preparing meals for one is understandably expensive; it also takes a little bit of willpower. However, there are ways in which the preparation and cooking can be made easier and not so costly. Although small freezers are expensive to buy, they are ideal for storing complete meals that only require defrosting, cooking or re-heating. Perhaps a quick telephone call the night before would remind the elderly person to remove the meal from the freezer in time to defrost. Alternatively a friend or neighbour could store meals in their freezer for your relative.

Problems with Diet

Spending a day having a 'cook-in' with your relative can provide an entertaining way of preparing a number of meals. Alternatively, economical meals can be prepared in a pressure cooker, slow cooker, the oven or one saucepan.

Easy Cooking for One and *Easy Cooking for Two*, both written by Louise Davies and published by Penguin Books, are excellent for people living on their own or for elderly couples.

If your relative is physically handicapped in some way, preparing meals can be very difficult; with a little ingenuity and some experimenting it may still be possible to preserve independence. Do not forget about the skills of the Occupational Therapist, who can advise on aids and new ways of dealing with household tasks. For example, try cooking vegetables in a chip basket, metal sieve or steamer to avoid having to pour off the boiling water. A shoulder bag or a basket hung on a walking frame makes it easy to carry a Thermos flask and food from the kitchen to the dining area; alternatively, a small trolley can be loaded with crockery, utensils and food and wheeled to the appropriate place. A liquidiser is the ideal gadget for the person who has difficulty in swallowing. The food tends to look uninteresting, but at least it is possible for the disabled person to have a complete meal.

Wholemeal bread sandwiches provide an ideal substitute for meals. The traditional meat-and-two-vegetables routine does not have to be followed when your relative cannot, will not or does not remember to cook or eat meals. The sandwiches can contain a variety of fillings and will constitute a balanced meal if eaten with fruit and milky drinks. The sandwiches can be prepared the day before and wrapped in a special cellophane wrapper to keep them fresh; in addition, if your relative is confused about the time, and may even forget to take the sandwiches, put an alarm clock beside the food and set it to go off at an appropriate time. By far the best method of encouraging an old person to eat is to have the meal together. If you can only call in once or twice a week, it's worth arranging those visits around mealtimes, so that you can reassure yourself that your relative is both able and willing to eat a reasonable meal, and one that can be enjoyed in company.

Making Use of the Services

If your relative is too handicapped or is reluctant to prepare meals, the WRVS 'Meals on Wheels' service can provide one cooked meal during the day. However, they are usually only able to function on five days of the week. Contact the local WRVS headquarters or the Social Services Department to enquire about the availability of the service in your area. In some areas frozen meals allow choice and a good meal daily.

Lunch clubs provide an excellent service to elderly people who live alone and for one reason or another are reluctant to cook meals for themselves; they not only provide a cheap meal, but a forum of activity and companionship. Some lunch clubs are part of large day centres for the elderly, while others are held in Church halls or local Community Centres. For those who are not club members friends and neighbours could arrange to meet in their own homes for a meal.

Inevitably, it is mainly the mobile, gregarious elderly who benefit most from the lunch club. Transport is provided by some clubs for the housebound and physically disabled, but for those who are mentally infirm and require a degree of supervision for an afternoon's stimulating activity there is little or virtually no support or provision, with the exception of day hospitals for elderly mentally infirm. If more transport were available and the 'lunch clubs' philosophy was extended to include activities for the mentally frail, more housebound and lonely people would benefit from such an excellent service. Why not lobby your MP or local councillor to improve or develop the services in your area?

6 Confusion in the Elderly

What is Confusion and why does it happen?

Everyone gets confused from time to time—confused about what to do next: feeling lost in a strange building: bewildered when you wake up suddenly in the night and for a split second don't know where you are. This feeling of confusion and bewilderment is usually short-lived. It is often associated with either unfamiliar surroundings, or conditions which give minimal information to tell us where we are, what time it is, or what we are supposed to do. Studies show that total sensory deprivation—when all information coming into the senses is shut off, for example by placing someone in a black soundproof room, with thick gloves and socks to cut off the sense of touch—quickly produces disorientation and confusion even in young healthy volunteers.

The problem may be the exact opposite—*too much* information for the brain to cope with. An example is the experience of getting lost in an unfamiliar shopping precinct on a busy Saturday afternoon, with a lot of noise, crowds of people pushing past you, and bright shop lights, but no clear indication of how you get in or out. This sort of experience is magnified when the brain has become either temporarily or permanently slowed up and unable to sort out with any certainty signals coming in from the world, or to make responses appropriate to those signals. Such are the sorts of difficulties and problems associated with severe confusion in the elderly.

The brain becomes more susceptible with age to the various causes of confusion for two principal reasons—loss of brain cells and a vulnerable supporting system that supplies the energy needs of the brain.

Cell loss in the brain occurs throughout life and once brain cells are lost, they cannot be replaced. This loss takes place at a faster rate as we get older. It occurs either through decay or through the failure of blood supply to small parts of the brain (so-called 'mini-strokes'). When these changes take place abnormally quickly, mental deterioration becomes evident in the form of Senile Dementia (Alzheimer's Disease) due to the rapid decay of brain cells, or Multiple Infarct Dementia, due to the cumulative effects of these mini-strokes. For most people this pattern of cell loss is sufficiently slow, and the number of brain cells remaining sufficiently large, that we automatically adjust to the slight reductions in mental functioning that occur with age.

The second reason for the susceptibility to confusion in the elderly is that the health and efficiency of other bodily organs become reduced with age; for example, as the heart and lungs become less efficient, they provide a poorer source of energy and support to the brain, contributing to its poorer functioning. Impaired functioning of other essential organs, such as the kidneys or liver, can also reduce mental efficiency.

In short, an increased susceptibility to confusion in the elderly results from age changes in both the brain and other organs in the body. The important role played by these other organs means that any serious physical illness can itself produce confusion in the elderly. In particular, any sudden development of confusion in an elderly person may very often be the result of physical illness outside the brain which, once recognised, can be easily and effectively treated.

How do you recognise Confusion?

If you are living with or looking after an elderly person, what should you look out for? There are a number of ways that confusion can show itself.

1. *Forgetfulness*—going out shopping and getting lost; mistaking or not recognising familiar people; confusion over dates and time of day; wandering at night; getting upset and muddled while carrying out everyday activities; losing the thread in conversation; forgetting words. There are very many ways in which increased forgetfulness can show itself. Such signs can be gradual and each 'mistake' on its own can seem insignificant, but month by month they may become more and more frequent in their occurrence. In contrast, obvious disorientation occurring quite suddenly may reflect not brain deterioration, but the effects of physical ill health—infections, heart failure, and many other illnesses can be responsible. If the underlying illness can be identified then the confusion can often be cured.

2. *Hallucinations and delusions*—the person may say he or she has been hearing or seeing strange, bizarre or menacing objects, people or animals. These 'hallucinatory' experiences may be more common in those with hearing or sight problems, or if the person lives alone. When they become linked to a fixed set of ideas—about prowlers getting into the house, or neighbours trying to drive them out of the

Confusion in the Elderly

house—they can form delusions of persecution which can be
stubbornly maintained even in the face of contrary evidence. Visual
hallucinations (seeing things which are not there) and transitory
delusions (irrational ideas which do not persist) are more commonly
associated with brain failure. Any persistent set of irrational beliefs (to
do with being persecuted, or having no money, or having some terrible
illness) is usually the result of a treatable mental illness, unconnected
with brain failure.

3. Wandering—the elderly person may suddenly wander off and get
lost, especially during a change of scene (moving house or on holiday).
While occasional signs of forgetfulness may have been apparent for
some time, the first upsetting sign of confusion is often when the
elderly person gets up in the middle of the night and starts wandering
about in the house, or even sets off down the street with no
explanation. Turning night into day is a common problem, especially
for those with persistent states of confusion.

4. Personality Change—associated with progressive confusion, and
sometimes the more obvious problem, is a change in the personality.
Growing indifference to emotional ties, a detached withdrawal from
everyday life and a coarsening of manners may occur early in
progressive brain failure. Concern for tidiness may be replaced by
increasing neglect of personal hygiene, behaviour may become
unpredictable, and emotional outbursts may sour relationships with
relatives and friends. While such changes usually occur in the
presence of forgetfulness and other signs of brain failure, they can also
occur because of a depressive illness. Depression does not simply
mean sadness and tears. Withdrawal, loss of interest, poor appetite
and poor sleep are often the main symptoms. Since depression is
treatable, it is important to alert your doctor if you detect these
changes in your elderly relative, rather than automatically assume that
they are part of 'senility'.

Persistent Confusion

Most commonly, confusion develops slowly and mental
deterioration cannot unfortunately be reversed. The medical diagnosis
of Senile Dementia, or Multiple Infarct Dementia, almost always
means that there is no hope of improvement in brain function.

Coping with Aging Parents

Deterioration will proceed, sometimes slowly, sometimes rapidly. In some ways this progression eventually makes life easier for the supporter. The earlier stages are often the most troublesome; with time, increasing brain failure leads to a quietening down. Care remains physically wearing, but the emotional drain seems to lessen. For some, this stage never arises, the wear and tear prove intolerable, and hospital or nursing-home care offers the surest relief. For others, the rather painful early conflicts and stresses pass; the older person may reach a stage of passive acceptance, and while the deterioration continues to be evident to those close at hand, it seems no longer to disturb or distress the elderly person.

How to Cope

There are almost no hard and fast rules. Each family is unique, each person unique. For some, the active maintenance of what mental abilities remain is important; for others, easing the passage through mental decline is the priority. The following suggestions may not always fit in with your own approach. The only rule of utmost importance is to have medical confirmation of the cause of confusion. It is not good enough to say 'It's just old age'.

First, the *physical environment* can be modified. If the elderly person lives alone, remember that tasks which require memory place a strain on the failing brain. Gas cookers and fires have to be turned on and turned off, lit and extinguished, and any inflammable material kept away from them. Electric appliances are generally safer. If you feel there is a risk of the person falling, make sure that no fire is unguarded; a guard that is fixed in place is essential. Get a kettle that switches itself off, and guards to prevent pans from being knocked over. Try to get a telephone installed if the person hasn't already got one.

Signs in clear bold letters may be a help. Too many 'memos' about the place may be too confusing but one or two clear reminders can help. Large clocks downstairs and in the bedroom (you need one with an illuminated face here) and a simple day and date calendar can act as reminders of the day and time of day. A card with your own telephone number and that of the doctor's surgery clearly marked, above the telephone, and a rail leading from the bedroom to the bathroom, with luminscent tape on the top can all help orientation.

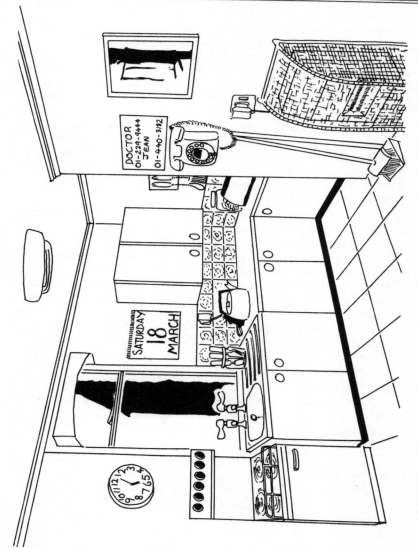

Make the environment as safe as possible, and put up a few clear reminders

Coping with Aging Parents

Finally, avoid clutter. A tidy, ordered household reduces the chances of people forgetting where they put things. As people get older they often accumulate more and more things in their house. Nevertheless the combination of personal souvenirs, essential clothes and bedding, tableware, crockery and kitchen implements should be kept to a minimum to remain homely, but reduce confusion. Some people label wardrobes and drawers as simple reminders of where things are.

If you live together as daughter, son, husband, sister or wife, then clearly you often have to be the memory for the confused elderly person. Helpful advice on this matter, is contained in a booklet entitled *Forgetfulness and the Elderly: How can you help?*, available from the Scottish Health Education Group, Woodburn House, Canaan Lane, Edinburgh EH10 4SG.

The second point is *communication* with a confused elderly person. There are several important points to bear in mind. Speak slowly; wait for replies; don't expect the person to grasp long sentences, with many different messages. Be patient, even if you're answering the same questions for the tenth time that morning. It's better for them to keep things in mind, than to give up altogether because of your frustration. Be tolerant when the elderly person is extremely forgetful—'Do I have a son? I don't think so . . .' Remember that memory failure can seem to destroy even the closest relationships, but that often recognition and memory will return, even if only in glimpses, fragments of the past. Allow the person to talk of the past—memories are often firmest then and provide a surer ground than the ever changing, poorly remembered recent events.

Be wise; when confusion produces distortions of the present or of the past, don't rush in to correct them. Sometimes it is better to ignore any 'crazy' ideas, rather than feel bound to criticise them for talking nonsense.

The third point is to *distinguish between the different forms of confused behaviour.*

Confusion can occur because the person misinterprets where he is, or who he is with; it may occur because speech centres in the brain are affected, making the person unable to say what he means, and producing jumbled, incoherent sentences. It may occur because the person has forgotten what he was intending to do, or had just done. It

Confusion in the Elderly

may also occur because those parts of the brain linking our actions together has been affected, so the person gets mixed up while dressing, or setting the table. Finally, agitation can aggravate, and sometimes actually cause confused behaviour. We must all have experienced being muddled as we rush for the train, or for an appointment, knowing we are going to be terribly late.

If the person is misinterpreting his surroundings, be calm; correct him, explain slowly where he is, use well-established cues to confirm 'reality' and try to remain matter-of-fact.

If the words sound confused and muddled, try and help by 'speaking for the person', to check that you know what he means. When possible, use objects or signs to make concrete what the person wishes to express.

If the person seems to have forgotten, try to think for him, and remind him what he was going to do; but do so in a matter-of-fact way. Suggest that he accepts his memory problems, and indicate that things often 'come back' when you don't try so hard. If the person is agitated and pressured by a sense of urgency that does not seem necessary, be firm and calm, and indicate that nothing is ever so important as to make us get into 'a state'.

Dressing and bathing are often problems for the confused person. If there is a problem with dressing, try to simplify the procedure. Lay clothes out in the order in which they are put on. Try to reduce the number of clothes in the wardrobe. Avoid complicated outfits with zips, buttons, and difficult fasteners; try to replace them with sweaters which can be put on 'back to front', skirts with elasticated waistbands, dresses which fasten up the front or which are simply got into without any buttons or zips at the back, sides or front. If a man has real difficulty with buttons and zips on his trousers, replace them with Velcro tape. Slip-on shoes are easier than those with laces.

If the person gets upset and anxious about bathing, try to develop a standard routine which fits in closest to their customary habits. Try to avoid arguments about whether or not to have a bath; deal with each step one at a time. Use only a few inches of water, and use non-slip mats on the bottom of the bath to reduce fears or unsteadiness. If you cannot manage, ask the district nurse to visit. Apart from the hygienic aspect, the opportunity to see the elderly person undressed alerts you to such health problems as rashes, sores and other physical ailments.

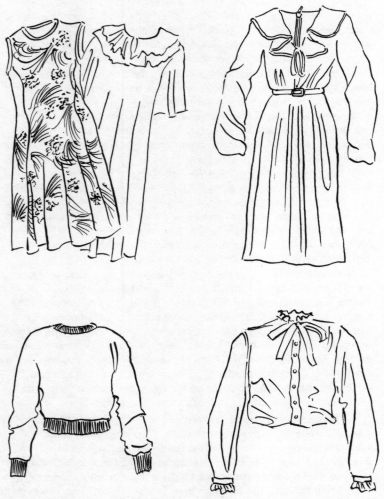

Easy-to-fasten clothes (left) are better than ones with fiddly buttons or zips (right)

Confusion in the Elderly

Of course all these hints may not always suit your own particular circumstances, and it is more important to act as you feel right than obey a set of rules which can never apply to all those unique circumstances that alarm, infuriate or even amuse. Confusion will show itself in different ways in different people. For some, it is a quiet, placid forgetfulness, for others an active, disruptive insistence on doing the wrong thing at the wrong time.

An active but confused person will not be satisfied cooped up in the house all day, but may need to be out and about, stalking old haunts, searching for old friends. You may be afraid of letting the person wander, even if you put a card with name, address, and your telephone number in a handbag, wallet or inside pocket. You may feel embarrassed going out, fearing some inappropriate remark or action by the confused person. Do remember that by the time we reach old age, as many as one in ten of us will develop severe forgetfulness and confusion. Most people are tolerant—shopkeepers will redirect the elderly person, policemen will take charge and contact you, passers-by will help if they see an elderly person at risk. You lose more friends through staying in, keeping the forgetful relative in the house and out of sight, than by visiting and risking the occasional embarrassing moments in friends' houses.

If your elderly relative seems confused, it is very important to get a correct medical diagnosis of the cause; it may be curable. But if you are having difficulties and your own doctor doesn't seem able to help you as much as you'd like, there are a number of organisations which can provide advice, counselling and other services. The *Alzheimer's Disease Society* was recently established to 'give support to families by linking them through membership; to provide literature to disseminate knowledge of the illness and also of the aids available through the Social Services to cope with it, and finally to see that adequate nursing care is forthcoming in the last stages'. See the chapter on Services, for details of how to get in touch.

Your local *Age Concern* offices may offer advice, and indeed may be running advice and counselling services to families in which there is a confused elderly person. Increasingly, day centres and day hospitals are being established to provide relief for families (or neighbours and friends) without the necessity of institutional care. It may mean you have to keep asking your GP or your local social services department, but it is worth getting the professional advice of those specially skilled in working with such people. Health visitors, community psychiatric nurses, geriatricians and psychiatrists can be relied upon to listen and advise on problems you may have.

If you feel you can no longer cope, or you need a break, it will usually be possible to have the elderly confused person admitted to hospital, sometimes for a fixed 'holiday' period. Some social services departments can also arrange 'holiday' admissions to a residential home for the elderly. Simply getting away, or getting out of the house alone, either to attend to your own business or just to relax a little is as important for the person being cared for, as it is for the carer. If your relative can go to a local authority day centre or specialised day hospital, this can free your time at home for one or two days per week.

One final word of caution. Because an elderly person seems at times to be confused, do not discount any wild story that he or she tells you. It may be true. Recently an elderly confused lady visited her daughter's house, and told her of a bearded young man who brought posters to stick all over her house. It was only later, at a meeting for relatives at the psychogeriatric day hospital, that the daughter realised that a doctor had indeed visited, and with the health visitor, had helped put up signs to remind her mother where her clothes were, and labelled the kitchen, bathroom and bedroom doors, to help reduce some of her confused wandering about the house.

Summary

1. Confusion results from both the environment and the brain's ability to cope with the environment. Any illness in the elderly may cause a temporary slowing of brain function, so that an environment which was once familiar and manageable becomes strange and confusing. The *sudden* appearance of confusion in an elderly person should always lead you to the doctor, for a thorough check of the person's physical health.
2. A sudden change in environment (moving house, or on holiday) can lead to the sudden appearance of confusion. Here, it is likely that a slow, previously unnoticed decline in the brain's abilities is brought to light by the challenge of the unfamiliar. Even if a return to familiar surroundings is possible, the confusion may remain in less acute form.

Confusion in the Elderly

Contacting the doctor at this stage is wise, but may not lead to any satisfactory 'cure'. Nevertheless, the doctor can be alerted to the possibility of mental decline, and you can be alerted to the need for advice and possible help in the future.

3. When confusion becomes a regular, persistent problem, you can help by being patient, being tolerant, being slow, and being practical. The more you can accept forgetfulness and confusion, the more reassuring you will be; the more you can help, in a matter-of-fact way, to correct mistakes, to supply lost memories, and to encourage as much independence as possible, the more the confused person can remain as little affected by his or her decline as it is possible to be.

4. Advice and help can be found if you need them. Services do exist to ease the difficulties of caring for the elderly mentally infirm at home. Services often come to those whose demand is loudest.

5. Share the caring. Whenever possible, try to enlist the help of neighbours, friends and relatives so that you can have a break during the day.

If you think of the mind as a flame in a candle, slowly reaching the end of the wax, then think of your help as hands round the flame, keeping out the stresses and upsets that could blow out the flame, but not so tightly that you are smothering it. Keep your hands just a little bit distant, so you do not get burned yourself. Emotional disengagement does not mean indifference, but it does mean learning to accept the nature of mental decline. The person who is slowly slipping further and further into mental oblivion will be less and less like the father, wife or sister you have known. This may be distressing, but it is necessary to accept the fact so that your care is based on both the memory of your relative and their present needs.

7 Problems with the Toilet

One of the greatest fears associated with growing old is that of losing bladder or bowel control, with the ensuing threat to self-esteem and independence. Using the toilet is regarded as a private matter, not to be discussed openly. At an early age we are taught to adhere to strict rules of toilet training. Not to do so is seen as socially unacceptable and can lead to punishment, ostracism and social withdrawal. It is therefore not surprising to find that incontinence in the elderly ushers in shame, guilt and fear. The elderly person who is aware of an incontinence problem may be mortified by his or her state. Help may not be sought and it may be only after a while that the problem is discovered by a relative who may find soiled underwear wrapped in newspaper below the bed. This is a pity since incontinence is best treated at an early stage. Many people, including professionals, believe that incontinence is synonymous with old age. This, of course, is grossly untrue. Incontinence is a symptom of a specific disorder which merits full investigation, treatment and management. No person, whatever his age, should suffer the shame and indignity of incontinence; nor should the carer be left to tolerate the stale smell of urine or basket-loads of laundry. It is not surprising that incontinence is often the last straw and may indeed be the chief reason for the elderly person being admitted to institutional care, simply because home support has been withdrawn.

The aim of this chapter is to describe the principal factors which can cause incontinence in an elderly person, and to outline measures that may alleviate some of the problems with the toilet. First, however, it is worth looking at the normal mechanism of passing urine and identifying some of the changes that take place in the urinary system of aging people. Approximately every 24 hours, the kidneys produce 1.5 litres (2½ pints) of urine comprising waste products, water and salts. Following its production, urine dribbles down two fine tubes called ureters and accumulates in the bladder for discharge. The act of passing urine is a reflex action and is caused by increasing pressure within the bladder. Because the conscious control of the passing of urine depends on the messages to and from the brain, diseases of, or injuries to, the central nervous system (of which the brain is part) are likely to affect this control. Moreover, with age, there are a number of bladder changes: for instance, its capacity may be reduced, it may not be completely emptied, or the desire to pass urine may be absent.

Problems with the Toilet

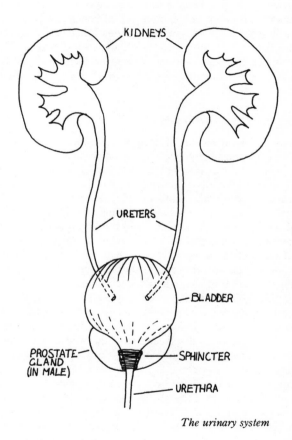

The urinary system

Coping with Aging Parents

The combined effect of these changes is that a person is likely to pass urine more often than previously, and possibly with little warning. The first condition is called frequency and the second urgency. Consequently the presence of one or more of these factors may lead to incontinence. It is not uncommon to find that these factors may be present in a person who remains continent, because the person modifies his or her lifestyle to meet these new demands. Therefore, if the carer has an understanding of these problems and takes measures to modify the environment, there is a good chance continence will be preserved.

Causes of Incontinence

There are many causes of urinary incontinence but broadly speaking they can be divided into two fairly distinct but inter-related categories: those which stem from physical and mental impairment and those related to adverse surroundings. Stroke, which leads to physical handicap, the pain and disability associated with arthritic conditions, Parkinsonism, ill-fitting shoes, ingrowing toenails, corns and bunions can all produce reduced mobility and thereby precipitate incontinence.

There are several other factors which can produce incontinence, e.g. infection of the urinary tract. This is characterised by a burning sensation on passing urine and leads to urgency and frequency. The prolonged wearing of rough and soiled underwear, and inadequate wiping after going to the lavatory may lead to infections.

Another disorder commonly associated with women is stress incontinence. It is a troublesome complaint due to weakening of the pelvic floor muscles or displacement of the womb after childbirth. It is characterised by spontaneous release of urine when laughing, sneezing, bending, coughing or lifting. Seek the advice of the GP, who may refer the elderly person to a consultant gynaecologist. In the meantime, suggest that the elderly person avoids situations which produce the symptoms. Also a pad may be worn to absorb any urine which leaks out. Sometimes, regular exercising of the pelvic floor muscles may relieve the symptoms. The physiotherapist could suggest the most suitable type of exercise.

Prostate enlargement and severe constipation are frequently associated with a condition known as retention of urine with overflow. Enlargement of the prostate gland produces a narrowing at the neck of

Problems with the Toilet

the male bladder which prevents the free passage of urine. Urine continues to accumulate despite the obstruction, but because the bladder is not being completely emptied urine tends to leak away in an almost continuous dribble. Severe constipation can also produce the same consequences because the large bowel and bladder are fairly close together.

The undetected diabetic whose symptoms include complaints of thirst and copious drinking may also develop incontinence.

Any tranquilliser, sedative or antidepressant drug may cause incontinence, especially at night when the elderly person does not have a full awareness of a full bladder or of the environment. Many falls have occurred when an old person has attempted to reach the toilet during the night. Commodes placed by the bedside and the presence of a dim light will help greatly to reduce the risk of night-time incontinence or falls.

Incontinence Resulting from Mental Disorder

Psychological disturbance caused by lifestyle changes such as the admission to hospital or residential home, the grief engendered by bereavement and loss and the anger and despair that result from frustrating situations are all capable of precipitating incontinence. Alternatively, for the elderly person who feels insecure and rejected, incontinence may provide an attention-seeking device, while for others it may be a means of protest. Severe depression can lead to a sense of giving up, with consequent self-neglect and incontinence.

More often than not, the person who suffers from dementia appears to be physically healthy but because of the pathological changes in the brain, the person may forget where the toilet is or may misinterpret something else as the toilet. He or she may not be able to interpret the feeling of a full bladder or remember the sequence of events undertaken to empty the bladder. The person may start soiling because the use of toilet paper has been forgotten. In all cases of incontinence, it is always prudent to have a full medical investigation to exclude infections or gynaecological problems; but where the cause is basically psychological, much patience and tolerance are required on the part of the carer to find the root cause. Thereafter, toilet training may well bring the desired continence.

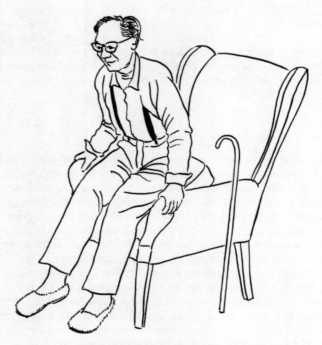

Special chairs are available which make it easier to get up

Problems with the Toilet

Environmental Causes of Incontinence

Even with the most thorough assessment and treatment of their disabilities, some elderly people are still unable to reach the toilet in time. It is particularly frustrating for a person who has adequate warning that he needs to go to the toilet, who is aware of the steps which he could take to prevent himself becoming incontinent, but is unable to take these steps because some feature of the environment prevents him. Rearrangement of the furniture may be necessary as well as a number of environmental modifications to make the journey to the toilet easier and therefore quicker, but firstly it is important to ensure the person can rise from the chair more quickly. The domiciliary occupational therapist or physiotherapist can be contacted via the Social Services Department and her first step will be to teach the person a new way of using the environment. If time is lost struggling to rise from a low easy chair, she may be able to teach them how to move to the front edge, place their feet and hands correctly and move easily and less painfully. If this fails, blocks under the chair will help and if this fails, a different chair may be the answer. The next step is to decide if ascent of the stairs and manoeuvrability in a toilet can be made easer by additional handrails or a raised toilet seat. Also the positioning and type of flushing system may influence independence. Alternatively, it may be worth considering installing a toilet and bathroom downstairs. If this step is to be considered, it is possible to obtain an improvement grant from the local authority. As mentioned in an earlier chapter, liberal signposting of the environment may help the dementia victim overcome incontinence although some may not be able to read notices. In such cases, a brightly coloured picture on the toilet door may give a helpful clue to identifying the correct environment.

Tackling Incontinence

The achievement of continence, or the management of incontinence, is possible by anticipating and avoiding the creation of some of the situations known to precipitate incontinence. However, this alone is not enough. Most importantly, the carer should adopt a sensitive attitude towards the elderly person for management to be effective. The need to take the total environment into account will also contribute to success. Reporting incontinence to the doctor is the first step. Remember, incontinence is a symptom of an underlying disorder and not an illness in itself to be associated with old age. Now assuming that certain investigations have been carried out—and these are more revealing than ever before, due to the setting up of urodynamic clinics in many areas—and the appropriate treatment prescribed, the carer may still be required to manage the problem. Firstly, ask the doctor, health visitor or district nurse to contact the occupational therapist who will advise on and arrange for the fixing of aids in the home. The district nurse can also give advice on special clothing and equipment; for instance pants are available which incorporate a small pad to absorb urine, or the use of Velcro fastenings to ease dressing and undressing; the Kylie bed sheet can absorb urine without its surface being wet; the use of a plastic urine bottle, or small urine dish for women or a commode may save much time and energy doing laundry.

The basic aim for incontinence management is to contain the urine. More recently, professionals have been advocating the procedure of toilet training. This involves three steps over a period of approximately three weeks:

1. Take the person to the toilet at intervals of about two hours spaced over the period in which incontinence is thought to occur.
2. Record brief details of the person's condition on these visits to the toilet, i.e. dry or wet.
3. To increase the capacity of the bladder to hold more urine over a longer period of time, visits to the toilet should be made every two hours and fifteen minutes. This may cause incontinence to return but this timing should be continued until continence is re-established.

When continence is reinstated for a period of 24 hours, an additional fifteen minutes is added and the process repeated by gradually increasing the bladder capacity. In this way the interval between toileting can be increased by increments of fifteen minutes every third day until a maximum of about three hours is reached. Whenever the incontinence chart reveals that the person is invariably wet when the time comes to visit the toilet, it may indicate he or she is not being taken early enough. In some instances, success may be achieved by moving the two hourly intervals backwards by an hour—even this may be too much of a time shift and it may be necessary to move the time backwards by fifteen minutes until such time as the person is found to be dry and then start again. It may be tempting to restrict fluids for the incontinent person, but this can make matters much worse by causing dehydration and confusion; however, it is sensible to give more fluid in the morning and less later in the day. Helpful hints on establishing such a toilet training regime are available in a booklet entitled *Management for Continence* published by Age Concern, or Dorothy Mandlestrom's booklet on *Incontinence*, published by the Disabled Living Foundation (see Chapter 2).

Faecal Incontinence

Like urinary incontinence, faecal incontinence should never be accepted as a normal process of aging. It warrants the same investigation and medical intervention, so do seek medical help if a relative encounters more than one episode of faecal incontinence. There can be many reasons for faecal incontinence but the most common cause in the elderly is constipation. The build up of very hard faeces in the large bowel irritates the lining, causing the production of excessive mucus which leaks past the hard mass. Your doctor should be consulted and he may ask the district nurse to give an enema. The nurse will also advise your relative to take a diet high in fibre such as vegetables, bran, cereal and wholemeal bread. Laxatives should be taken with care and again the doctor or nurse will suggest the most appropriate. This is discussed in more detail in the chapter on Diet.

The smearing of faecal matter over clothes, furniture and walls can be the most distressing form of incontinence to deal with. This type of problem can be associated with mental impairment and is probably the most difficult to tackle. However, if you follow the same guidelines as are described for urinary incontinence, i.e. thorough medical examination and treatment, avoidance of constipation with a diet high in fibre and liquids, continence should be preserved. The offensive smell commonly associated with incontinence can be avoided or dealt with by the immediate immersion in cold water of soiled garments and bed linen. Also, effective deodorants can be obtained from the chemist.

The symptom of incontinence, which is sometimes referred to as the 'thief of self-respect', has been regarded as an inevitable consequence of old age for far too long. Any steps that might be taken to restore continence, or to minimise the effects of incontinence, are therefore worthy of serious consideration. Do not be afraid to seek advice from the GP, the health visitor, district nurse and local social service department.

8 Problems Through the Night

Looking after an elderly person can become very trying when your sleep is consistently disturbed. We all need sleep to recover from the physical and mental exertions of the day. When an elderly person has to be attended to at frequent intervals throughout the night, their demands can begin to seem overwhelming, and as patience and energy wear out, so conflicts at home can multiply. Getting a good night's sleep is important both for the person being cared for, and for the person providing the care; it will restore energy and relax the mind in preparation for the inevitable demands of the day.

With age it seems that there is less need for sleep, perhaps because less mental and physical energy is used during the day. This leads to an overall reduction in the time spent asleep at night, a generally lighter type of sleep, and more frequent awakenings during the night. These three changes are gradual, and in themselves should not prove cause for concern. Unfortunately many elderly people— used to habits of early bedtimes and early rising because of work—fail to realise the natural changes taking place in their sleeping pattern, and fret over lying awake at times when, in the past, they would have been sound asleep. This is no doubt one reason why the over-65s are the most frequent users of sleeping tablets.

The physiological changes that alter sleeping patterns with age also have other consequences. They can make the elderly person considerably more vulnerable to night-time disturbances, particularly in the presence of physical or emotional illness. Many old people do enjoy their sleep, accept the changes in their sleep pattern with equanimity, and do not develop physical or emotional illness. A significant minority are not so fortunate. For them, the sleep pattern becomes seriously disrupted. Four major factors are most often responsible for such disruptions—mental infirmity, bladder problems, physical ill health, and emotional problems. We will deal with each of these in turn.

Confusion

By no means all confused elderly people have disturbed nights; such people are, however, particularly prone to sleep disturbances. The degeneration of brain cells which accompanies mental deterioration in old age produces an exaggeration of the changes in the sleep pattern brought on by age—sleep is shorter, lighter, and broken more often than in normal elderly people. During these periodic awakenings, the brain is less capable of correctly interpreting the surroundings and judging what is happening.

In the dark, there is less information to go on. If someone suddenly wakes you up in the middle of the night, it takes some time before you can fully comprehend what is happening. For the mentally infirm, this loss of orientation is greater and much harder to recover from. The mentally impaired person's senses may more easily deceive him. The imagination is less effectively checked by logical thinking and may give rise to fears which then serve to intensify the confusion.

At other times, waking in the night may lead to behaviour normally associated with waking in the morning. There may be good reason for waking, and for getting up during the night, but with a failing memory, such reasons can quickly be forgotten; the elderly person may find himself up, but not able to remember where he is, what time it is and why he is out of bed.

How to Help

Confused and disturbed night-time behaviour often results from poor information, or mis-information, in the dark; there are several ways of alleviating this problem. If there is a dim night light, the elderly person can more easily make out where he is, should he awaken. Leaving the bathroom door open, and the light on, can also provide an easily identified locator which may be needed during the night. A large illuminated clock, placed in a clearly visible position, may reduce the risk of mis-interpretation of the time. A clear and uncluttered pathway to the bedroom door can reduce the risk of falls.

Inactivity, both physical and mental, can reduce the need for sleep. Elderly and mentally infirm people are less able than most to generate their own activities. A certain degree of mental and physical stimulation during the day will often ensure a better night's sleep. For example, relatives often report that after visiting a Day Hospital, or Day Centre, their elderly dependent sleeps more soundly that night.

Drinks that stimulate the brain (and bladder) should be avoided late in the evening. Tea, coffee or fruit juices should not be given; a bedtime drink of warm milk, milky cocoa, chocolate or Horlicks is better if you hope to induce a good night's sleep.

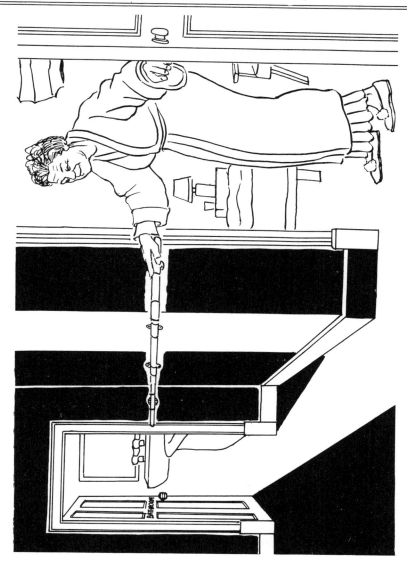

Make it easy to find the bathroom at night

Coping with Aging Parents

If confused night-time behaviour has become such a problem that drugs are being used, it is worth remembering that over-sedation can reverse sleep patterns; the elderly person may sleep during the day and remain awake at night. Normal sleep patterns can often be re-established by reducing sedation, or discontinuing it altogether (with the doctor's approval). If sedative tablets are prescribed, do not assume that an increased dose will ensure sleep. This could be highly dangerous. Keep the pills out of harm's way, for a person waking confused in the night may easily take an extra one by mistake. Always check with your doctor about pills, and dosages. Ask him whether any of the pills your relative is getting could contribute to disturbed sleep.

How you handle night-time problems is important. Learn to avoid lengthy conflicts, struggles, and commotions, and to handle such incidents as do occur more quickly and more effectively, so that both your own sleep and that of your relative is least affected.

Night-time wandering is the most frequent problem; it may be lost, aimless wandering, or agitated and driven. The former is easier to handle. Remind the person where he is, what time it is, and who you are. 'It's two o'clock in the morning, Father, you don't need to be in the hall. Come along with Jenny, now, I'll help you back to the bedroom. You can have another five hours sleep yet, before you need to get up. Do you want to use the toilet?' Provide, in a calm, matter-of-fact way, all the necessary information to help re-orientate the person and check on any important problems. This kind of reassurance and orientation should help to reduce further confusion.

The second type of night-time wandering can be more difficult. The elderly person seems distraught, and has some obvious purpose in getting up. He may believe that prowlers are outside the house, or that someone is calling his name, or that it is time to go to work. A mistaken belief, based on imagined sounds or sights, can be accompanied by considerable emotional distress, ranging from anger to terror. Under these circumstances it is better to spend some time with the person, before getting him back to bed; deal logically with his problems; correct, calmly but clearly, any misinterpretations; and, if need be, offer to check out the matter further in the morning. When the person has become less upset, it will be easier to persuade him to return to bed. Spending a little time ensuring that he is comfortable in bed—showing concern, plumping up pillows, and smoothing out sheets—can help him to settle back to sleep.

Problems through the Night

Although such disturbances are extremely demanding, and although patience is extremely thin at two o'clock in the morning, taking a few minutes extra to give cues, to calm and correct the confused person can be worth it; it will reduce the likelihood of agitation and further disruptions during the night. In addition, the more effectively you feel yourself coping, the less likely *you* are to become disheartened by the demands of caring.

For the elderly person who lives alone, night-time wandering, especially outside the house, can provoke alarm and anxiety in neighbours and relatives. It can be even more disturbing when the elderly person blithely denies any such behaviour the following day. Sometimes it can be helpful to alert the local police, who could patrol the area, and keep an eye out for anybody wandering about.

The police can be a valuable source of help in other emergencies. An elderly, stoutly built gentleman fell out of his bed one night, while his wife was in the bathroom. She could not lift her husband back to bed, nor could he manage himself. After a telephone call to the local police station, two burly constables soon arrived, and gently lifted the old man back into his bed. In other circumstances, the police may be willing to stop during their regular night-time patrols, to reassure an elderly person who is spending his nights in fear of prowlers. The reassuring voice and sight of the local policeman can be a great source of comfort to many elderly people who live alone.

The Bladder

Most elderly people need to get up two or three times during the night to empty their bladders; there is also less time available between feeling the need to go to the toilet and the bladder actually emptying. This in turn can lead to anxiety, and a fear of wetting oneself, which can itself serve to disrupt sleeping patterns. Certain practical measures can, however, be taken to avoid accidents.

1. Drinking enough. At least four or five pints of liquid daily, with less consumed in the evening, will prevent dehydration, reduce the likelihood of constipation, and prevent infections of the bladder. It is a mistake to reduce liquids, as adequate fluid intake helps to protect against bladder infection.

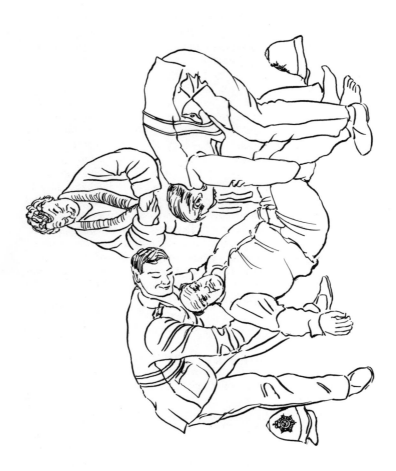

2. Developing greater control during the day. By exercising the muscles responsible for emptying the bladder, holding on for longer during the day, and building up the bladder's tolerance for 'feeling full', the night-time intervals between visits can be extended, thus reducing the amount of disruption to sleep.

3. Daily Vitamin C may help prevent urinary tract infections, which can cause an increased need to go to the toilet, and occasional 'wetting' episodes.

4. Easy access from bedroom to toilet. A bedside commode with lift-down arms can be recommended when it is clearly too difficult—for reasons of physical infirmity—to reach the toilet at night. But if the person can, with help, reach the toilet, it is better to have handrails fitted from the bedroom to the bathroom, to assist them. This has the advantage of encouraging and maintaining independence. In a shared bedroom, the one with the greatest need should sleep nearest the commode or bedroom door!

Sudden changes in bladder habits (especially the development of incontinence) should always lead you to consult your doctor. Remember that certain disorders can produce incontinence. These include diabetes, prolapse of the womb and enlarged prostate gland. Incontinence can also be caused by some types of pills.

If night-time incontinence occurs in a mentally infirm person, it is harder to correct, and is less often due to treatable conditions. However, the possibilities of 'toilet training' are sometimes worth trying. More details of this are contained in an Age Concern (England) booklet, *Management for Continence* by Bob Browne. Information on incontinence aids, such as pads, pants and special sheets can be found in Chapter 2.

Physical Illness

Any illness is likely to disrupt the vulnerable sleep of the elderly person, by causing inactivity, pain, discomfort, anxiety and isolation. Although sleep is a valuable aid to recovery, the lack of activity imposed by illness can make it harder to come by. These days it is realised that complete bedrest is rarely necessary, and indeed can serve to *impede* recovery from illness. After checking with your doctor that it is safe to do so, try to encourage the person to spend some time during the day up and out of the sick bed. Even sitting in a chair beside the bed can be a help, doing relatively undemanding physical exercises; reading, writing letters, or solving crossword puzzles can equally exercise the mind. A companion, ready to talk and listen, to chat or play cards, is not only a source of mental exercise, but an ally to dispel the worries that illness calls up in so many of us, young and old. Such efforts will generally be repaid with a sounder night's sleep.

Pain, discomfort or breathlessness can be a torment. Even with these physical symptoms, a caring and reassuring approach can have its healing effects. Sitting with the person in the evening, playing some favourite music, reading a well-liked book or some poetry, plumping up the pillows, smoothing out bedclothes—all such demonstrations of care can actually help to reduce physical suffering, and can bring about the necessary relaxed state of mind for sleep.

Worries about illness and fears of going to hospital, or even dying, can produce sleepless nights. This may make the invalid very demanding—calling out for water, aspirins, help to go to the toilet, and so on. Relatives may often feel that the invalid is 'putting it on', demanding attention and enjoying the 'sick' role. We must all have done this, at one time or other—capitalising on others' sympathies. Nevertheless, appropriate and regular care and attention during the day, and being allowed to talk over any worries—no matter how irrational they may seem—will make it less likely that nights are disrupted by fearful, attention-seeking requests.

Finally, when ill health combines with mobility problems, and you cannot lift the person to the toilet at night, it may be possible to call upon night nursing services, who can visit once or twice during the night to lift and toilet the elderly invalid. Such services can be requested from your local GP, although they are not always available. Another aid which may prove useful in cases where the elderly person sleeps alone is the Care Call alarm system. For some elderly people, the need to get out of bed can pose problems, and you may fear that he may fall and hurt himself without your being aware of it. The Care Call system provides a sensor device, placed under the foot of the bed, with an extension lead to an alarm unit which will indicate, either through a warning buzzer or a flashing red light, when the elderly person leaves his or her bed. In addition, there is a call button system, so that the elderly person can summon help when you are in another room. See Chapter 2 for details.

Problems through the Night

Another way of providing effective communication at night is a two-way 'intercom' system (such as can be obtained from Mothercare shops), which can cut down the amount of anxiety felt by both the carer and the cared for, and prevent unnecessary journeys to and fro between rooms.

Emotional Disturbance

Anxiety and depression are likely to affect sleep, whether in the old or young. Sleep may be harder to come by, or may be disrupted and difficult to regain. Insomnia can become a chronic problem in its own right. A very high number of people aged 65 and above regularly take sleeping tablets. Night-time sedation carries with it considerable risks for the elderly, and should be sought only when there are extreme difficulties, and then for only short periods of time.

Confusion, falls, nightmares . . . there are many unfortunate consequences of over-sedation. Some of these disadvantages are more thoroughly covered in the chapter on 'Medicines'. If your relative complains about sleeping badly, and if you suspect that he is also becoming more withdrawn, irritable, or preoccupied with health or money problems, it is worth encouraging him to visit the doctor as this may be an early sign of depression. Perhaps, however, he is already taking sleeping tablets, but feels they are 'not working'. Sometimes there are practical ways to help, without pills.

Older people sleep less, and do wake more often—this is a fact to be accepted, not fought against. Too early to bed, and then hours spent awake, will be no help. Setting a later bedtime, doing some light reading, or other relaxing occupation, having a warm milky drink before retiring, can all help. Taking more exercise during the day, building up gradually and slowly to a more active day time routine, can also increase the need to sleep.

Loneliness can be especially acute at night. If your elderly relative lives alone, an evening chat on the 'phone can be very helpful and reassuring. It may be possible to arrange a regular system of evening phone calls, with other members of the family, or friends, so that the caring can be spread more evenly. If the elderly person does not have a telephone, it may be possible to have one installed under the Chronically Sick and Disabled Persons Act—see your local social work/services department.

Night Hospitals

There seems to be a strong case for 'night hospitals' to be established, on the same lines as day hospitals, so that particular problems at night can be eased by allowing the elderly person to spend some nights during the week in hospital, to give the carers a little relief. While day hospitals and day centres exist in many areas, there remains a gap in the health and social services to supplement family care over the night-time period. Perhaps, with appropriate encouragement, the authorities will in the future consider such schemes as night hospitals, extending the already valuable services of day hospitals and day centres, and easing the demands on those people who are trying to keep their relatives at home for as long as possible.

9 Medicines for the Elderly

One leading expert on medical care of the elderly recently wrote that 'prescribing in Britain today is in a mess'. Almost three-quarters of the population over the age of 75 are receiving one drug or another, but there is a widespread feeling that a large number of these prescriptions are both unnecessary and potentially harmful. One of the biggest problems associated with prescribing drugs for elderly people is that unwanted side-effects are more common and may lead to poorer rather than better health. One in ten hospital admissions for the elderly are attributed directly or indirectly to the unwanted effects of drugs which have been prescribed for them.

The various organs of the body tend to become less efficient with increasing age; the way these organs handle, absorb and eliminate drugs may also become less efficient. This process can lead to the unwanted accumulation of the drug and its by-products so that levels of concentration in the body are reached which produce harmful rather than beneficial effects. On top of this, elderly people often take several different sorts of pills at the same time and are thus at risk of getting mixed up over what to take, when and how often. The answer is, of course, not to throw away the drugs, but to develop a more careful and responsible attitude toward their use.

Many elderly people take their medicines without any problems or complications. There are no muddles, no untoward side effects, no misunderstandings of instructions. The general aim of this chapter is simply to alert carers to the potential hazards that can arise and to suggest ways of making sure that all those elderly infirm people looked after at home are kept as free as possible from such hazards.

Common Categories of Medicines

If you are looking after an elderly person with any degree of infirmity, one of the most important things is to be familiar with any medicines or pills that he or she is taking, whether on prescription or bought over the counter from a chemist.

The list that follows describes the types of drugs used for disorders affecting the various organs and systems of the body, together with some of the more commonly used prescriptions.

The heart and circulation

Anti-hypertensives: drugs like methyldopa (Aldomet) which are used to reduce high blood pressure.

Diuretics: drugs like frusemide and thiazides (Lasix and Navidrex-K) which help the kidneys to get rid of excess fluid which can build up due to a poor circulation and weak heart.

Cardiac stimulators: drugs like digoxin (Lanoxin) which help stimulate the heart in conditions of heart failure.

Drugs for irregular heart beat and angina: drugs like propranolol and metoprolol (Inderal, Betaloc) which help reduce irregularities in the pumping action of the heart. They are also used to treat angina (chest pain due to constrictions in the arteries of the heart).

The chest and respiratory system

Bronchospasm relaxants: drugs like salbutamol (Ventolin) aimed at reducing tightness in the chest and breathing difficulties associated with asthma, bronchitis and emphysema.

Expectorants: drugs like bromhexine and promethazine (Bisolvon, Phenergan) which help to ease congestion and are used to treat dry coughs.

Antibiotics: drugs like ampicillin (Penbritin, Ambaxin) aimed at killing off bacterial infections of the chest and respiratory tract.

Muscles and joints

Anti-inflammatory agents: drugs like indomethacin and ibuprofen (Indocid, Brufen) that help to reduce the pain and swelling associated with arthritis, rheumatism and other disorders of the joints. Less commonly used are steroid preparations like prednisolone (Prednesol) used to treat some forms of rheumatism.

Analgesics: drugs like aspirin and paracetamol used to treat pain associated with a wide variety of conditions including inflammatory disorders of the joints and muscles.

Stomach, bowel and bladder

Antacids: drugs containing aluminium and magnesium salts to treat indigestion, gas, heartburn and hiatus hernia. Some antacids contain sedatives to relieve tension and spasm as well. Gaviscon is an example of the former, Aludrox SA of the latter.

Medicines for the Elderly

Laxatives: drugs to treat constipation (Dorbanex, Isogel).
Anti-diarrhoeals: includes straightforward anti-diarrhoeals such as Kaolin mixture and drugs containing an antibiotic (Kaomycin) when diarrhoea is due to an infection.

Nervous system

Anti-convulsants: drugs like phenytoin and phenobarbitone.
Anti-depressants: drugs like amitriptyline and mianserin (Tryptizol, Bolvidon) used to treat depression and anxiety.
Anti-Parkinsonian: drugs like levodopa and benzhexol (Sinemet and Artane) used to control the rigidity and tremor associated with Parkinson's Disease.
Hypnotics: drugs like nitrazepam and triazolam (Mogadon, Halcion) used to treat insomnia or sleep disturbance. Barbiturates such as quinalbarbitone (Seconal, Sodium Amytal, Soneryl) were once widely used, but most doctors agree that these tablets are habit-forming and potentially *very dangerous* if taken in overdose.
Tranquillisers: There are two groups—the minor anxiety-relieving drugs like diazepam and chlordiazepoxide (Valium, Librium); and the major tranquillising drugs like thioridazine and promazine (Melleril, Sparine) used for the relief of more severe agitation and mental disturbance.

This grouping of drugs and the various bodily systems they work on is not meant to be by any means comprehensive. It is a broad outline of many of the compounds prescribed to elderly persons. What is important for you, as the carer, is that you have a clear idea of what tablets or syrups the person you care for is taking, and the reason for the medicine. If he or she is taking more than one type of medicine, you need to be aware of what possible problems might arise, and to know which medicines are the most important ones. Any changes in medicines should be understood and any possible problems arising from the change should be explained. If necessary ask the doctor, and if you don't trust your own memory, get the doctor or pharmacist to write down what you need to know. You don't need expert knowledge, but if you are responsible for the administration of medicine to an elderly infirm person, you have both the right and the duty to know what medicines you are taking care of.

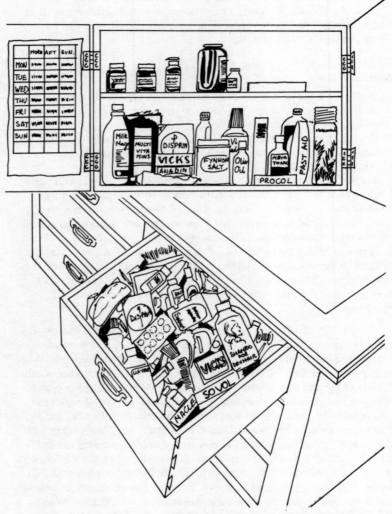

For safety's sake, drugs must be stored tidily

Medicines for the Elderly

Keeping Tabs on Tablets

Older people see more of their doctors, as a general rule. It follows that they are thus more likely to receive medicines. Bottles and boxes with illegible names stored amongst letters, packets of pins, and over-the-counter medicines, can make it difficult to take the right pills, in the right order, at the right time. If you are not in daily contact with the relative you are caring for, you may well worry about the number of pills they take, and the risks of confusion. Following the guidelines set out below will help.

1. Make sure you have a clear idea of what medicines are in the house, and make sure that pills and syrups are discarded once they are no longer being used, or have passed their expiry date (particularly in the case of 'over-the-counter' medicines). Every few months make a point of listing all the medicines, and if it seems an awful lot, take the list to your doctor and check with him.

2. Keep all medicines in one cupboard, on their own, and in a safe place. If you feel the person you look after is prone to get confused, or is absent-minded, then store the main containers and the daily doses *separately*, so that large quantities cannot be taken by mistake.

3. Make sure all labels are clear and readable—the name of the pill or syrup, the dosage, and instructions on taking them. You can ask your local pharmacist, GP or district nurse to arrange special large-print labels, or special plastic tags.

4. Make sure pills are accessible—child-proof containers and small-necked bottles stuffed with cotton wool can be impossible for elderly people with stiff joints, or restricted power in their fingers, hands and wrists to manage. Some older people find wing-cap dispensers easier to use than screw-on caps—talk to your local pharmacist or district nurse if you think this is a problem.

5. Keeping a record card, as a check and reminder of pills to be taken, can be very helpful. Using stiff 6″×4″ cards, you can write down the time, medicine, what the medicines are for, the dose and a check (✓) for when the medicine has been given. The example overleaf shows what such a card could look like. Such cards provide a record of what medicines are being taken, and will be a handy reference for visits to the hospital or surgery. If kept in the medicine cabinet, cupboard or drawer they also serve as a reminder. They help

MEDICINE RECORD CARD

TIME	MEDICINE	WHAT FOR	DOSE	S	M	T	W	T	F	S
7.30 am	Ampicillin (black and red capsule)	Chest infection	1 tablet	✓	✓					
12 noon	Ampicillin	Chest infection	1 tablet	✓	✓					
4 pm	Ampicillin	Chest infection	1 tablet	✓	✓					
10 pm	Ampicillin	Chest infection	1 tablet	✓	✓					
	Nitrazepam (white tablet)	Sleeping pill	1 tablet	✓	✓					

build a routine which maintains the best 'timing' for taking pills. Finally, they provide a brief explanation of why the pills are being taken.

If you do not live with the elderly person, the card can be filled in by the district nurse, if you can arrange for her to call and administer the pills on the days you cannot visit. The doctor, health visitor or district nurse can help you make out such cards, and advise you on this sort of record-keeping. Some elderly people can be encouraged to keep such record cards themselves, but they need help to begin with and ideally community nurses should be involved in providing that initial guidance.

6. Alternatively, you can buy 'easy-open' clear glass containers, and put each day's dose in the container. For example, if pills are taken in the morning and evening, you will need two containers for each day, one labelled 'MORNING' and one 'EVENING'. If you visit at weekends, then you can set out the week's medicines, or three day's medicines, and a home nurse/district nurse can do the same mid-week. We have even seen clear plastic egg-boxes used as a way of 'dispensing' the right tablets!

Such problems as forgetting or getting confused will quickly be identified, and this may point to the need for more supervision—you may find, for instance, on Saturday that Thursday and Friday morning's medicines have not been taken. On the other hand, when there are dozens of tablets in a bottle, it is very difficult to know whether they have been taken.

Medicines for the Elderly

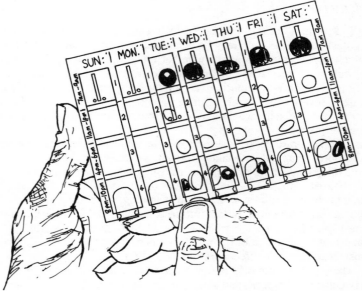

Dispenser box for pills

Through the chemist or district nursing sister, it may be possible to get Dosett or Medidos tablet boxes; these are divided into 28 sections, four sections for each day of the week, each section labelled with a time (e.g. 8-10 pm). The box can store a week's prescription, and can be used by the elderly person him- or herself. However, no elderly person should just be left to get on with this system. It is very important that getting used to using these dispensers is accompanied initially with help, advice and checking.

7. Make a periodic search to ensure that no old medicines are lying around anywhere. Don't allow *any* medicines to be hoarded or forgotten.

This may sound like a lot of work. It certainly requires some effort to be so conscientious about pills, but it really is worth it. Modern medicines are both powerful and potentially dangerous, if misused for any reason.

Medicines and Side Effects

Side effects are those produced by a drug, which are additional to the desired effect. They may be beneficial, e.g. the sedative effect of some antidepressants: they may be harmful, e.g. the irritant effect of aspirin on the stomach. The problem increases in older people. These side effects can vary from the very minor ones, such as a dry mouth, to quite severe effects which can be potentially fatal. It is as well to be alert to the problems which may arise from the administration of drugs to older people.

To take a rather extreme example, the following side effects have been noted from patients taking the anti-hypertensive drug, methyldopa: sedation, drowsiness, transient headaches, depression, nightmares, impaired mental alertness, dizziness, light-headedness, spasms, swollen ankles, weight gain, vomiting, constipation, sore tongue, fever, anaemia, nasal stuffiness, swollen abdomen, dry mouth. These are by no means certain or even likely to occur; it is still important to be aware of the problem and to ask the doctor what the most important side effects are to look out for.

Many paradoxical effects can occur with drugs—sleeping tablets may actually *disrupt* normal sleep patterns, while some tranquillisers may increase agitation and produce added confusion. Pills for blood pressure and heart disorders can produce emotional side effects such as depression. Medicines bought without a prescription, such as pain killers and cough medicines, can also create problems. It is important (a) if the doctor or hospital prescribes new tablets, or changes the dose of medicines, to ask if there could be any side effects to look out for; and (b) if there is any sudden change in the health or behaviour of the person you are caring for, to check whether this has followed any recent change in medication.

The message is simply this—share the responsibility of caring with the professionals. Don't be afraid to ask, and make sure you understand what you are told. Only through such partnership can the best care be given.

Over-the-Counter Medicines

Many people habitually buy medicines direct from the chemist for minor aches and pains, colds, tummy upsets, and disturbances of the

Medicines for the Elderly

bowels. It is not sufficiently recognised, however, that such medicines often carry their own risks. For instance, decongestants may increase heart rate and blood pressure, especially in the elderly with circulatory problems. The drying agents in some cold remedies can influence the pressure within the eyes, which is potentially dangerous for those with an already existing problem of raised pressure (glaucoma), and can lead to further worsening of vision.

Many antacid preparations contain sodium salts, which can be harmful to people on a low salt diet because of high blood pressure. Milk of magnesia is probably one of the safest medicines to give to an elderly person with an upset stomach, since it does not contain any sodium salts. Aspirin can irritate the stomach lining, and cause ulcerations and bleeding— especially if taken in excess. Anaemia can develop in the elderly after long-term use of pain killers such as aspirin, as a result of slight but persistent internal bleeding. Excessive use of laxatives can lead to dehydration, and impair the normal functioning of the bowels.

Proper food, sleep and daily exercise remain the best means of maintaining health for all of us. If you have any worry that the person you are looking after is over-zealous in the use of such over-the-counter medicines, have a word with your doctor. This simple precaution could save you a lot of trouble.

If you are responsible for administering *any* medicines, then take that responsibility seriously. You don't have to be a doctor or a pharmacist, but you do need to know what medicines you are handling and why. As a carer you have the right to work with the professionals, and to share responsibilities and information, to achieve the best possible form of caring.

10 Personality Conflicts

Caring for people with some degree of disability or infirmity is not just a question of looking after a body. Both the carer and the person cared for have many conflicting feelings and thoughts to contend with. We do not take on the role of carer overnight. Recognition of the transition from a pre-existing relationship of husband, wife, daughter or sister to one of carer is usually a slow process. For some people it may not seem like a change at all—simply an extension of care and concern for your partner's or parent's welfare. Inevitably, however, the task of providing long-term care does bring about changes in the relationship and with those changes come problems and conflicts which can make the physical and practical demands of caring much more burdensome. This chapter deals with some of the conflicts that can arise from the caring relationship.

The Responsibility of Caring

For some relatives the biggest problem is simply deciding whether or not to take on the job of providing care and especially whether or not to accept an elderly infirm relative into your home. This step is often taken without thinking through the consequences. For many people it is the right decision but it is enormously important that the heart should not dominate the head in weighing up the situation. Ask yourself the following questions:

What disabilities does the person have, and what can be expected for the future? Don't hesitate to seek advice from the doctor and social worker.

How much can you reasonably give to the care of that person? Most of us are neither physically nor emotionally equipped for total self-sacrifice. Be quite clear what responsibilities you wish to take on, what others around you will give, and what support you can expect from the social and health services.

What might be expected of you by your relation? Can you agree together on how much independence each should have? If you start out giving all the time, how easy will it be if the rewards of giving become overshadowed by the burden of caring? Do you feel bound to be entertainer, companion, nurse and financial advisor and is this really necessary? It is better not to exhaust yourself early on and thus be able to find more energy as the caring role expands.

Personality Conflicts

Do consider the value of sharing the responsibility early on, before beginning what is really a career in caring. Arranging for the whole family to discuss such a move will help to clarify how much responsibility you can expect to bear if you do decide, with others' advice, to take your elderly relative in to live with you.

We will discuss the idea of family conferences and the use of professionals in advising and supporting carers in detail in Chapter 11.

Changing Positions

Probably the most frequent change in roles is that experienced by sons or daughters who, having throughout their lives been accustomed to some form of parental support, now find themselves in the position of being called upon to give support to their parents. The adjustment required from almost automatically seeing your parents as pillars of strength, to seeing them as individuals increasingly dependent upon you, is considerable and may even prove intolerable.

This problem of adjustment is, however, not one-sided. For many elderly people there can be considerable unease about becoming a 'burden' on their children, and also a less consciously acknowledged anxiety about transferring their position of 'looking after' children, to being themselves the ones who are looked after. For some elderly parents, this change carries with it all sorts of fears of dependency, loss of self-esteem and personal weakness. Few of us pass through life without doubts about ourselves and our ability to cope with life's demands. Such hidden fears may be released by the growing awareness of our reliance upon 'our children.'

Another common problem arises from attempts to transfer one style of relationship onto another. This may be seen, for example, after an elderly man is widowed, when he seeks from his children the same unconditional caring, concern and sympathy he had from his wife. The children, however, may have grown up believing that their mother too often 'gave in' to father, and from this different perspective they may feel quite determined to avoid such indulgence and not permit themselves to be 'oppressed' in the way they feel their mother was. The result could easily be feelings of resentment on their part and of abandonment by the father, who believes that his children show no real interest in him.

Coping with Aging Parents

Becoming a Child Again?

A related problem is seen in an exaggerated style of caring for an elderly person where the carer (often a daughter), stresses the person's disability and gives excessive 'mothering' care. This has been called 'infantilisation' of the elderly. The role of carer is very close to that of a parent and it is understandable that the woman, perhaps at a time when she is relinquishing her role as mother to her own children, reproduces that pattern with her elderly parent.

But the reversal of roles is not exact; we expect to see our children growing up, and encourage their growing independence, telling them not to be 'childish'. In the altered circumstances of caring for our own parents, we may omit this element from our caring/parenting role. We do things *for* the older person, not with them. We focus our communications on their 'dependency', not their 'independence'.

'How are you feeling now?' we may ask, subtly strengthening our expectation of ill-health and infirmity. We do the cleaning, cooking and shopping for our mother. We dress and undress her, rather than help her dress and undress herself. Instead of helping to maintain a sense of personal responsibility we may foster dependence: rather than shopping *with* her, or deciding with her what shopping to get, we go out and shop *for* her. Similarly when making a meal, rather than deciding *with* her what to make, or even making the meal with her, we do it *for* her. Often, the reason is given that it's not practical, or it just creates problems and arguments. Unquestionably it is more difficult and time-consuming to involve the elderly person in such activities. However, even the arguments and discussions help the elderly person to maintain a sense of independence and responsibility, and it is important that no one wins all the time.

Occasionally such infantilisation takes on a quality of parental bullying. The elderly person's attempts to do for himself/herself are brushed aside: 'Here, let me do it: you can't manage that'. Their capacity to be independent is minimised, and their dependency is exaggerated and enhanced, as if to emphasise how helpless they are. Hidden behind such efforts at caring may lie considerable hostility and anger. Attempts at exercising independence may be quickly criticised, and excessive efforts made to emphasise what the elderly person cannot do.

A further motivation toward infantilisation can be found—a

desperate attempt to be needed and loved. One middle-aged lady would come home from her twice-weekly visits to her mother filled with anger and sadness. After bringing in the coal, collecting and taking away the washing, cleaning, shopping, dusting and cooking, she still felt she could not elicit the recognition and love she desperately needed. Throughout her life, from childhood onwards, she had felt unloved and unappreciated by her mother. Yet she alone of her sisters and brothers continued to work hard at earning this love and affection. Each time she failed, her anxiety and guilt (for maybe she didn't love her mother either?) fuelled her energy and efforts to be a caring daughter—increasing her frustration and pushing her mother further and further into apathy and dependence.

Changes in Marriage

One problem frequently faced by husbands and wives is a shift in responsibilities when one partner develops some disability. If a husband has been relied upon to look after the bills, do jobs around the house, and seek his own friends and entertainment, the onset of disability may result in a dramatic shift in responsibilities. Inactivity, and a reduced ability to take decisions and manage household repairs, may prove frustrating to him and frightening to his wife, who feels herself suddenly having to do things which had always been taken care of by her husband. She may resent him being 'under her feet', and find him a silent and unresponsive companion.

Alternatively, if the wife has become disabled, the husband may find himself saddled with unaccustomed household chores—feeling he is doing 'women's work', and resenting or finding it difficult to cope with these new demands. It is not uncommon for men to have relied upon their wives to develop and keep up social contacts and friendships, and when the wife is no longer so independent, social isolation may quickly surround both partners.

Sexual problems must not be ignored. In some cases growing mental infirmity may make the sexual act a source of anxiety, if not repugnant to the other partner. Alternatively, physical disability may make intercourse extremely difficult if not impossible, leading to sexual frustration. Sexual feelings are not absent in elderly people, but it is useful to remember that sexual needs include tenderness, the need to hold and be held, and the need for physical demonstrations of affection. If the act of intercourse is impossible or unpleasant for one partner, it should not become a reason to avoid any physical demonstration of affection and closeness. However, the couple should not feel embarrassed to discuss major sexual problems with the doctor. If sex is a worry—either because of its absence or excessive presence—it may help to talk over these problems.

Setting the Limits

Whatever the past history of the relationship between 'carer' and 'cared for', it is unlikely that we can resolve historical conflicts by finding new motives for our caring. We should rather try to define the limits of the caring relationship as clearly as possible. For some elderly couples, the memories of a shared life create a sense of unconditional acceptance of whatever responsibilities caring should bring.

This marital solidarity (for such feelings are found most often, though not exclusively, in husbands and wives) may ignore the changes brought on by physical or mental infirmity in one's partner. Indeed it may seem as if life itself is engulfed by the role of caring, that your purpose in life is governed by the responsibility of looking after your spouse 'till death us do part'. The more able partner may indeed feel guilt that while he/she has escaped many of the problems of aging, the other has not. The predominant feeling may be one of sadness, as the caring partner sees how old age together has been transformed from mutual sharing to single-handed caring.

Such unlimited concern is not to be criticised, but it does create problems. People often fail to recognise the demands that are being placed on themselves and their own health, and fully to appreciate the needs of their partner, and the degree of change and disability he/she has undergone. Although it may be painful, and sometimes induce a sense of guilt, the opportunity to step back from such 24-hour caring, to 'disengage', is worth taking even if it leads only to a conscious acceptance of continuing to care as before.

For others, the responsibility of 24-hour caring may not be accepted so willingly. The experience of being trapped in the role of carer, of seeing your life narrowing down further and further, may lead to resentment and then guilt over such frustrations.

The irritation and frustration of feeling trapped in the caring role

Personality Conflicts

may serve to build up further resentments, and further guilt. Disabilities observed in the elderly infirm person may be misinterpreted as deliberate attempts to gain attention and make life more demanding and restrictive. Such behaviour may evoke hostility, which in turn alternates with guilt, keeping the carer from any attempts to take time off and to escape for a while from the task of caring. This may then lead to resentment towards other family members, who come to be seen as 'leaving it all to me'.

For children, the problem of limits may arise because of a sense of divided loyalties. Responsibility to parents conflicts with responsibility to your own partner, and your children. It may seem that you are torn in so many different directions, that in the end each attempt to satisfy one person only produces anxiety about neglecting the other. This sense of feeling pulled in different directions is often unavoidable, but the opportunity to step back, to decide what the limits are, should always be taken.

Can We Avoid these Conflicts?

So far we have been concerned with identifying the various conflicts that can arise in determining the personal relationship between carer and cared for. What practical steps can be taken to minimise these problems?

It is unrealistic to expect human nature and personal relationships to be capable of straightforward solutions. Sometimes the only alternative to caring is simply giving up, accepting that you have reached the limits and seeking some institutional long-term care. Sometimes it is enough to have a good friend to 'sound off' to, someone who can recognise that caring also produces resentment, anger and frustration. On other occasions, practical help is the best solution—perhaps arranging for the elderly person to attend a day centre or day hospital, or arranging for some other member of the family to share the responsibility by looking after your relative while you have a holiday, or coming in one day a week to help. It may be possible to arrange a voluntary sitter, or holiday admission in hospital, or in an Old People's Home.

Yet again, it may be necessary to take stock of what disabilities the elderly person has, what limitations he/she has, and how dependent he/she in fact is. A health visitor or occupational therapist, as a professional outsider, may help give you a clearer picture of what needs the person has, and how best you can meet them. The Crossroads Attendants scheme may help to provide a flexible service so that you can take a break from caring. Details of this scheme to provide a sitting service for carers can be found in Chapter 2.

Taking a break such as a short holiday can sometimes make it easier to recognise how much strain you are under. It is a mistake to feel that you should never give up. No one can be superman or superwoman, and rationing your caring is neither selfish, cruel, nor disloyal. If physical infirmity leads to growing restrictions on what the person you are caring for can do, it is important to appreciate what the limits on your own health are, and to decide how much to do for them. When mental infirmity leads to a gradual loss of the person you once knew as husband, wife, mother or sister, it is necessary to accept that change, with inevitable sadness.

By recognising as honestly as possible what limits you have and what limitations your elderly relative has, you can best judge how much help you need. By sharing the task of caring, you do not limit your feelings of care, but allow them to be expressed in their most effective way, freed from resentment, anxiety, frustration and guilt. If you can only visit once a week, then by accepting that limitation you can make that visit more pleasant, more constructive and more effective. By arranging to leave your husband or wife once or twice a week—with a friend, volunteer, day centre or day hospital—you do not 'desert' them, but give yourself freedom and relief so that you can conserve both the physical and the emotional energy necessary for caring. By openly expressing your frustration and anger to someone else you can go a long way to avoiding such feelings creeping into the everyday acts of caring. Remember— caring for others involves caring for yourself.

11 Continuing to Care

Sometimes a family is unable to care for an elderly frail person at home, even if relief services are available. The task of caring can be a 24-hour job, and may require the skills of a professionally trained person. The decision to place your elderly relative in a nursing home or a hospital can be difficult to make, and it often takes time. Frequently families have tried everything else first. However, a time may come when institutional care becomes the most responsible decision the family can make.

Great sadness, grief and guilt may be felt at having to accept the inevitable decline of a spouse, parent or sibling. Frequently there are mixed feelings about the decision; a sense of relief that care will be taken by others, yet at the same time feelings of guilt for wanting someone else to take over the real burden. Anger may also be felt because there is no other choice available. Many people do not want to place their elderly relative in a home or hospital, they feel they should carry on the care at home because they do not want to be seen as 'dumping' the old person in an institution. In fact most families do all they can to postpone or prevent admissions, and after admission they visit on a regular basis.

There is a tendency to imagine that in bygone days all families took care of their elderly at home. The truth is that few people lived long enough for their families to be faced with the burden of caring. People who did become old and sick were in their fifties and sixties and the sons and daughters who cared for them were very much younger. Today many children of an ailing parent are themselves in the fifties and sixties.

Making the Decision

It is not unusual for family members to disagree about institutional care. Some may want the elderly person to remain at home while others feel the time has come for him or her to enter a hospital or home. Misunderstandings and disagreements are often worse when everyone does not have all the facts, and it is helpful if all involved family members discuss the problem together in a family conference. Sometimes the doctor or social worker can join in to help clarify the aims of the discussion. We suggest you follow three basic principles when organising a family meeting:

1: Everyone attends who will be affected by the decision.

2: Each person has his or her uninterrupted say.

3: Everyone listens to what the others have to say, even if they don't agree.

If there is misunderstanding or disagreement about what is wrong with the elderly person or about how to manage future care, it may be helpful to ask the doctor to explain these issues. It is also important to talk about financial issues. It may seem insensitive to think of such things when an old person is sick, but they can be the underlying cause of much bitterness.

To contemplate giving up the care of your elderly relative at home and handing over that care to an institution must surely be one of the most difficult decisions of a lifetime. Inevitably it will cause heartache. No one can tell you exactly what to do or make that decision for you; there are no right answers. Each person is unique; what is right for one person is wrong for another, and only you can make the decision.

Anger and frustration are normal responses to caring for a person whose behaviour is difficult. However, when your anger begins to affect your relationships with people and when you take your anger out on the old person it is time to take stock.

Do not be afraid to ask for help. Sometimes sounding off to a friend or a professional—doctor, health visitor or social worker—can relieve the situation, but it can also indicate that you need to make a decision about future care. Ask yourself these questions:

Do I feel that I am out of control of the situation, or at the end of my tether?

Is my body telling me I am under too much stress?

Do I feel panicky, nervous or frightened?

If the answer to these questions is yes, you may be carrying too heavy a burden and the time may have arrived for you to decide upon the transfer of your elderly relative to a home or hospital.

Choosing the Right Type of Care

Many elderly people live alone, but for some their independence is jeopardised by physical and mental infirmity. Friends, neighbours and family may consequently become alarmed and frightened at the prospect of a continued independent existence at home. If you have made sure that all possible resources have been mobilised to help the old person to remain at home, and yet there is still a risk to their safety and health, the GP and/or social worker should be contacted and asked to put the wheels in motion for a move into a residential home. However, do discuss with your relative your own concern over their welfare living at home and then inform them of your intention to contact the professionals. As mentioned earlier, this can take a long time; much depends on the area in which you live and the resources available.

Another determining factor is money. When there are large sums of money available, private nursing home care can be considered.

Before any arrangements are made for the move into continuing care, the doctor will determine the nature of the problem. For instance, if your relative is suffering from a severe degree of dementia, cannot dress himself, is incontinent and wanders aimlessly, he would be referred to the psychogeriatricians for placement in a psychiatric hospital. Alternatively, if the elderly person is not confused or only mildly confused, is able to wash, dress and is continent, placement would be considered in an old peoples' home run by the social services department or a voluntary association.

Placement in a geriatric hospital or nursing home is determined by the degree of physical infirmity. Sadly, there are insufficient resources to cater for the growing number of elderly people who require continuing care, which means that the carer sometimes has to carry on with their burden for much longer than originally anticipated. Nevertheless, where an old person's circumstances worsen, the GP or social worker should be contacted to hasten admission.

Applications for admission to privately-owned and voluntary organised homes can be made by a relative, but applications for a local authority residential home have to be made through the social services department. Once application has been made, a social worker will visit the applicant to discuss the need for residential care and to assess suitability and the degree of emergency. She will bring an application form to be completed with information about present and past circumstances and family, in addition to physical condition (for instance, hearing and sight) and how independent the person is. Other questions will concern business and financial aspects of the old person's life, in particular a statement of financial circumstances, including information on pensions, savings and whether or not the home is owned.

This information is required so that the local authority can assess how much to charge for residence. The elderly person must sign the form before the social worker can start to look for a placement. Generally, once a place has been offered it has to be accepted or rejected within a few days. However, it is usually possible to visit or arrange an overnight stay in the unit prior to admission. Do not be too hasty to give up a home until you are sure your relative is settled.

Making the Move

Understanding something of what the old person may be thinking and feeling may help make the move easier. The move may mean giving up independence and admitting disability. It means giving up a familiar place and familiar possessions which are the tangible symbols of the past, and reminders when memory fails. No old person should just be uprooted and 'dumped' in a home or hospital. Take steps to involve the person as much as possible in plans for the move, even if he is reluctant to go. He is still a person, and his participation in plans and decisions that involve him is important unless he is too severely impaired to comprehend what is happening.

Old people who have been hoodwinked into a move may become angry and suspicious, and their adjustment to the new setting may be extremely difficult. When a person is too impaired to understand what is happening it may be better to make the move without the added stress of trying to involve him in it.

Changes can be very upsetting to old people; no matter how carefully you plan the move, this is a major change and the person may be upset for a while. After a period of adjustment he will usually settle into his new surroundings, but occasionally an old person never really adjusts to moving. Don't blame yourself; you did the best you could and acted for his well-being.

Adjusting to a New Lifestyle

The move into a residential setting can be very painful for the cared for and the carer. Adjustment takes time and energy, but the move does not necessarily mean the end of your caring. Your relative is still part of the family and there are many things you can do to make the adjustment easier.

For instance, if your relative is suffering from dementia you can help orientate him to the new setting. While visiting you can explain the daily routine. Show him where the bathroom, toilet, dining room and lounge are. Help him find his things in the wardrobe and think of a way to identify his belongings and furniture as his own. Use photographs and ornaments to remind him of the family. Encourage him to remain a part of the family by keeping in touch with events such as birthdays and anniversaries, provide him with a notebook or diary in which you can record the special events together. If he is not seriously ill, involve him in outings, a walk around the grounds, a visit to a nearby teashop or a visit home for the afternoon. Sometimes you may feel able to manage him at home overnight but if you do, discuss the proposal thoroughly with the staff. Talk about the family, the neighbours and gossip, take with you tape recordings of the children or of people who cannot get in to visit.

Help him to care for himself. Bring in a treat which you can eat together, or if your relative has difficulty in eating, visit at mealtimes and help to feed him. Encourage your own children to visit, but before they do, explain to them the things they are going to see.

Sometimes people are too ill to be able to communicate verbally or even to recognise you. It can be hard to know what to say and you may feel it is not worthwhile visiting. Your visits are still important and although you may not be able to entertain or actively participate in caring, it is sufficient to sit and hold hands, or talk quietly and calmly about the day's events.

Disengaging

It is usual for families to feel lost, tired and guilty for a while after their loved one has been admitted to residential care. It may be difficult to decide what to do or to relax enough to watch television or read, or even to sleep the whole night through.

Visits to your relative may be tiring because of the distance you have to travel and possibly because of the depressing nature of the other residents. The move may have intensified your feelings of loss and grief and you may wish you could have carried on caring for the person at home. You may have mixed feelings of relief, sorrow, guilt

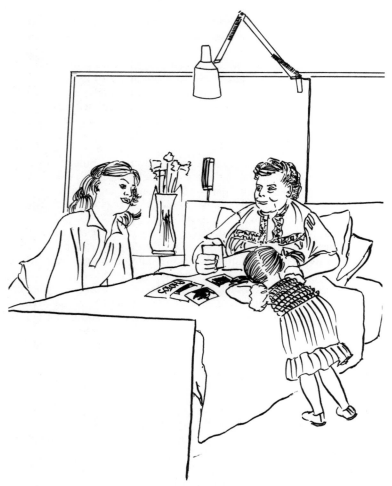

Help your relative to remain part of the family

and anger. Eventually you must acknowledge that it is a relief not to carry the burden and to get a good night's sleep or carry out a leisure activity uninterrupted.

Staff in the institution are trained to provide care for a number of people and there may be times when you feel your relative is not being cared for as you would like. There may be other things that upset you; for instance, your relative may not have had a shave or had his hair combed, or his clothes may be food-stained. If you are feeling angry do not keep things to yourself; you have a right to discuss these issues with the staff, to be given answers, and you will not jeopardise your relative's care or status in the home by doing this.

Although you may be a regular visitor, other members of the family and friends are not. This may be because they find it difficult to know what to talk about or they cannot face being with many frail, old people. If someone in your family reacts this way, try to understand that it may be their way of grieving. Alternatively, you could suggest that they visit with you, and make the visit very short.

Only you can decide, in consultation with the staff, how much time you spend visiting. Some relatives spend many hours visiting; this may have something to do with loneliness and grief. It may be better to spend less time there, so that the old person can make an adjustment to their new home. It is important to start making a new life for yourself, renew old friendships, take up a new hobby, buy some new clothes or organise a short holiday.

Mutual Support Groups

It is a common experience to feel that you are the only one who is suffering from the grief, guilt and anger associated with your relative moving into institutional care. This is far from true; many people share the same experience, as you will soon realise by talking to other relatives. To formalise and encourage a system of mutual support, groups have been formed in a number of homes and hospitals.

Meetings are informal, and usually take place once a month. The group discusses the issues involved in having a relative move into care and ambivalent feelings the carers have in 'letting go'. It is important that staff members are present to answer questions about the routine daily activities, the person's progress and some of the problems the staff inevitably encounter.

This means of communication and support can put relationships between staff and relatives on a much better footing. In addition, relatives and staff feel that they are working together to give a quality of life to the elders' remaining years. Many other institutions, especially hospitals, would benefit greatly if relatives could band together to organise fundraising activities, outings and the purchase of furnishings. If there is no such support system in your relative's home, why not suggest to the staff that one be set up? Alternatively, do not be afraid to seek help on an individual basis with a social worker or the person in charge.

When Your Relative Dies

Although your relative may have been ill for some time, and you may have expected death to occur long before it did, the event still comes as a shock.

Dying is an inescapable part of living, yet few of us discuss our emotions and reactions to dying before we are actually confronted by the death of a loved one. For some, death may be the release from a torturing illness, both for the person and the carer. It can also be the end of a protracted 'living bereavement', as experienced by carers of dementia sufferers.

If the death occurs at home, a doctor must be called. He has the responsibility of issuing a death certificate. If he has not seen the person for more than 14 days, the coroner must be informed of the death. If the death occurs in hospital, the doctor in charge at the time of death will issue the death certificate.

The next step is to register the death at the office of the Registrar of Births, Deaths and Marriages within whose boundaries it occurred. The law requires you to register a death within five days in England and Wales, and within eight days in Scotland. A copy of the entry and a disposal certificate, and one free copy of the Certificate of Registration of Death is given to the person registering it. A small charge is made for any extra copies needed when making insurance claims or settling the estate. The death cannot be registered if an inquest is to be held.

At this point it is usual for an undertaker to take over the arrangements for the funeral. If the body has to be cremated, note that the certificate has to be signed by *two* doctors; there are also forms to be completed before the cremation can take place. The undertaker will advise you on all matters connected with the funeral.

Funerals are quite expensive affairs and it is wise to ask for a written quotation. You can apply for a Death Grant by taking the death certificate, the marriage certificate (if applicable) and the estimate to your local social security office. The grant is paid on the basis of national insurance contributions of the deceased or those of the widow or widower, and is made to whoever is responsible for the funeral expenses.

The Death Grant is currently £30 but if the deceased was 77 years old (if a woman) or 82 years old (if a man) before 5 July 1975 then a reduced grant of £15 will be made. Additional help with funeral expenses can be obtained through the social security office if you are receiving supplementary benefit. If you cannot afford to pay for a funeral, the local authority can arrange a simple ceremony and claim the Death Grant themselves.

Bereavement

After the funeral there will be other matters to deal with, such as insurance, bank accounts, the Will, and so on. If you need help, Age Concern or the Citizens' Advice Bureau can provide it.

One of the most difficult tasks will be the sorting out and disposal of the dead person's belongings. The desire to hold on to the last physical evidence of their life is understandable. At this stage many bereaved people become very depressed, and convinced they could and should have done more to help. It is very important for the whole family to help anyone suffering in this way; in cases where the depression persists medical help may be needed.

To 'work through' the experience of bereavement, it is most important that feelings of frustration, fear and anger are given expression. The temptation is to repress them for fear of shocking or hurting family or friends. This repression can bring on sleeplessness, withdrawal, depression, loss of weight and abandonment of normal activities.

Most people find the first six months after bereavement are the worst. After this, the threads of life are generally picked up again. The final step in the process of grieving is when the dying, the death and the grief have been accepted, interpreted and absorbed into your life.

Coping with Aging Parents

This process can bring about positive changes in your personality. All life experiences help to develop the 'self'; bereavement can be one of the most influential and should not be regarded as a negative experience.

The emotional and physical strain of caring for an elderly infirm relative can be immense, but for most carers the task is an expression of love, accepted without resentment and carried on until the death of the old person.

A single woman of 60 had spent 15 years of her life caring for both disabled parents. She recalled with a tinge of sadness the missed opportunities to visit friends abroad and to further her career, but then, with a warm smile, she described the pleasure and privilege of being able to give love and affection. 'I know' she said, 'that they would have done the same for me.'